Benzodiazepine Dependence, Toxicity, and Abuse

A Task Force Report of the American Psychiatric Association

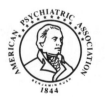

Published by the
American Psychiatric Association
Washington, DC

NOTE: The contributors have worked to ensure that all information in this book concerning drug doses, schedules, and routes of administration is accurate at the time of publication and consistent with the standards set by the U.S. Food and Drug Administration and the general medical community. As medical research and practice advance, however, therapeutic standards may change. For this reason and because human and mechanical errors sometimes occur, we recommend that readers follow the advice of a physician directly involved in their care or the care of a member of their family.

The findings, opinions, and conclusions of the report do not necessarily represent the views of the officers, trustees, or all members of the American Psychiatric Association. Each report, however, does represent the thoughtful judgment and findings of the task force of experts who composed it. These reports are considered a substantive contribution to the ongoing analysis and evaluation of problems, programs, issues, and practices in a given area of concern.

The paper used in this publication meets the minimum requirements of the American National Standard for Information Sciences—Permanence of Paper for Printed Library Materials, ANSI Z39.48-1984.

Library of Congress Cataloging-in-Publication Data

Benzodiazepine dependence, toxicity, and abuse.

    Includes bibliographical references.
    1. Benzodiazepine abuse. 2. Benzodiazepines—Physiological effect. 3. Benzodiazepines—Toxicology. I. American Psychiatric Association. Task Force on Benzodiazepine Dependence, Toxicity, and Abuse.
[DNLM: 1. Benzodiazepines—pharmacology. 2. Drug Utilization. 3. Prescriptions, Drug. 4. Substance Dependence. QV77.9 B4785]
RC568.B45B46 1990   616.86   90-571
ISBN 0-89042-228-1

British Cataloguing in Publication Data

A CIP record is available from the British Library

Contents

Preface

THIS TASK FORCE REPORT was prepared with the cooperation and assistance of a large number of people. Carl Salzman, M.D., Chairperson of the task force, served as primary author and editor. Portions of the report were also written by Mitchell Balter, Ph.D., Karl Rickels, M.D., J. Christian Gillin, M.D., Everett H. Ellinwood, Jr., M.D., David J. Greenblatt, M.D., and Roland Griffiths, Ph.D. Other members of the Task Force who provided critical comments include Donald M. Gallant, M.D., Herbert D. Kleber, M.D., Leo E. Hollister, M.D., Steven M. Paul, M.D., Edward Sellars, M.D., Ph.D., Charles P. O'Brien, M.D., Ph.D., and Robert C. Nelson, Ph.D. Harold Alan Pincus, M.D., of the APA Office of Research, provided considerable input, and Sandy Ferris of the APA Central Office provided patience and support. Seemingly endless revisions of the manuscript were cheerfully prepared by Elizabeth A. Quimby. Additional suggestions were supplied by Malcolm Lader, M.D., Eberhard Uhlenhuth, M.D., Markku Linnoila, M.D., Ph.D., and David V. Sheehan, M.D. The Chairperson wishes to express his grateful appreciation to all. No funds from the pharmaceutical industry were used in the preparation of this report.

Carl Salzman, M.D.
Chairperson

1

Introduction

BENZODIAZEPINES are among the most widely prescribed medications in the world. Well-established therapeutic uses in psychiatry now include treatment of anxiety, insomnia, and panic disorder. Less well-accepted therapeutic indications include treatment of depression, augmentation of neuroleptic treatment of schizophrenia, and symptomatic treatment of neuroleptic side effects. In other areas of medicine, benzodiazepines are used for anesthesia, to relax muscles, to treat seizures, and to calm anxiety and agitation that may be associated with illness. The popularity of these drugs derives from their high therapeutic-toxic ratio: compared with other sedative/hypnotic drugs, they are effective and relatively safe (Salzman 1988, 1989).

In recent years, patients, lay publications, and consumer groups (Bargmann et al. 1982; Brewin 1978; Cant 1976; Ehrlich 1988a, 1988b; Gordon 1979; Public Citizen Health Research Group 1987) have expressed concern about whether these drugs are overprescribed, although media reports may not always provide a balanced presentation of drug use (Hollister 1980; Lasagna 1980). Psychiatrists, in turn, have raised questions about the potential for these medications—especially some of the newer, high-potency, short half-life compounds—to produce serious side effects as well as to induce drug dependence (Ashton 1984; Carney and Ellis 1987; Cohen 1987; Herman 1988; Peet and Moonie 1977; Ramster et al. 1987). These concerns prompted the American Psychiatric Association to convene a task force to review the potential hazards of benzodiazepine use.

This task force report is not a comprehensive review of the pharmacology of benzodiazepines, nor is it a guide to their therapeutic indications and use. Rather, this report provides clinicians with a review of the available information on the potential hazards of benzodiazepine treatment and offers suggestions for the rational

1

prescription of these medications, when their use be clinically indicated. The specific goals of this report are listed below.

1. To review patterns of prescribing and clinical use of benzodiazepines.
2. To identify patterns of risk for the development of physiological dependence, especially at therapeutic doses; to examine whether or not there is a clinically important difference in risk of physiological dependence among the various benzodiazepines; to characterize the discontinuance symptoms that may occur as a result of such dependence; to suggest steps for the prevention and treatment of benzodiazepine dependence; to review pharmacological factors that cause benzodiazepine dependence.
3. To describe the acute and chronic toxicity that may result from benzodiazepine administration at therapeutic doses as well as at high or toxic doses; to identify risk factors among patients that may contribute to toxicity.
4. To examine patterns of benzodiazepine use outside the context of medical practice, such as the occasional use of unsupervised therapeutic doses for symptom relief; to examine use for recreational purposes as well as use as part of a poly–substance abuse pattern.
5. To place the above information in a clinical context; to enable psychiatrists to weigh the relative benefit versus the risk of using benzodiazepines; to identify factors that may increase the benefit and reduce the risk of their use; and to develop prescribing guidelines for the clinically appropriate use of benzodiazepines in clinical practice.

2

Clinical Pharmacology
of Benzodiazepines

I N THIS CHAPTER we will briefly review three aspects of benzodia-zepine pharmacology: 1) effects in the central nervous system (CNS), 2) pharmacokinetics, and 3) development of tolerance.

Effects of Benzodiazepines in the
Central Nervous System

Benzodiazepine derivatives are presumed to exert their pharmacologic effects via interaction with a class of high-affinity specific binding (recognition) sites, termed the benzodiazepine receptor. The binding sites for benzodiazepines are an integral part of the receptor for the major inhibitory neurotransmitter γ-aminobutyric acid (GABA). Benzodiazepines bind to the benzodiazepine-GABA receptor complex, enhancing the effect of GABA to hyperpolarize (decrease excitability of) neurons, thus enhancing CNS inhibitory tone.

Pharmacokinetics

The principal determinant of the extent of receptor occupancy is the absolute drug concentration in systemic plasma. Likewise, the time-course of receptor occupancy is completely dependent on the time-course of whole brain concentrations, which is in turn dependent on the systemic pharmacokinetic pattern of distribution, elimination, and clearance (Miller et al. 1987b). There is no evidence to indicate that any benzodiazepine "lingers" at the receptor longer than would be expected, based on its disappearance from plasma and from the brain.

Benzodiazepines may be divided into two groups depending on their biotransformation. Drugs in one group undergo several metabolic transformations that produce active metabolites, each of which has its own kinetic properties. An example of a drug with multiple step biotransformations is chlordiazepoxide, which produces the following clinically important active metabolites: desmethyl chlordiazepoxide, demoxepam, desmethyl diazepam, and oxazepam. These metabolites are considered "active" because they produce both therapeutic as well as toxic effects. Another benzodiazepine in the group that undergoes multiple step biotransformation is diazepam, which produces the clinically important metabolites desmethyl diazepam, temazepam, and oxazepam. Flurazepam produces the active metabolite desalkyl flurazepam. Other drugs in this group, such as halazepam, clorazepate, and prazepam, all follow the diazepam metabolic pathway (Table 1).

The second group of benzodiazepines does not undergo multiple step biotransformation and does not produce active metabolites. Examples are lorazepam, oxazepam, and temazepam. (Alprazolam and triazolam produce an active metabolite that is clinically unimportant.)

As a group, the benzodiazepines that undergo multiple metabolic steps accumulate gradually and are cleared more slowly from the body. The elimination half-life (half-life for short) is the time it takes for the concentration to fall by 50%. The active metabolites of these drugs also have their own elimination half-lives, usually $\geq 30\%$–50% longer than the parent compound. Thus, for example, the

Table 1. Benzodiazepine prescribing characteristics

Category, generic name	Trade name	Usual Daily dose (mg)
1. Long half-life, high therapeutic potency		
Clonazepam	Klonopin	0.5–4
2. Long half-life, low therapeutic potency		
Chlordiazepoxide	Librium	15–40
Diazepam	Valium	5–40
Halazepam	Paxipam	60–160
Prazepam	Centrax	20–60
Clorazepate	Tranxene	15–60
Flurazepam	Dalmane	15–30
3. Short half-life, high therapeutic potency		
Lorazepam	Ativan	1–6
Alprazolam	Xanax	1–4; 4–6
Triazolam	Halcion	0.125–0.5
4. Short half-life, low therapeutic potency		
Oxazepam	Serax	10–120
Temazepam	Restoril	15–30

average elimination half-life for diazepam in a healthy young adult who does not drink or smoke is 36–48 hours, whereas the elimination half-life for its active metabolite desmethyl diazepam averages 48–72 hours. In elderly patients these elimination half-lives are often doubled or tripled because of diminished efficiency of hepatic biotransformation.

As a group, benzodiazepines that are more rapidly cleared from the body are known as short or (short to intermediate) half-life drugs. These drugs accumulate in the blood less extensively but more rapidly than the long half-life benzodiazepines, and they are also cleared more rapidly (half-life is 14 hours or less).

In clinical practice, the term *elimination half-life* is sometimes confused with duration of action. The onset and duration of action of a benzodiazepine is related to its absorption, uptake into the CNS, and binding at the benzodiazepine-GABA receptor complex. For single dose or very short-term administration, the principal determinant of the onset of action is the rate of absorption and lipid solubility (penetration of the blood brain barrier). Thus, a long elimination half-life drug such as diazepam actually has a very rapid onset of action because it is rapidly absorbed and easily penetrates the blood-brain barrier. The duration of effect of a single dose of a highly lipid-soluble drug such as diazepam is also rather short, despite its long elimination half-life. Because of its lipid solubility, it rapidly redistributes out of the CNS (very much like a short-acting barbiturate anesthetic). In contrast, a short half-life benzodiazepine such as oxazepam is slowly absorbed, slow to penetrate the blood-brain barrier, and remains in the CNS longer than diazepam when given in a single dose. Despite its short half-life, the duration of action of an individual dose of oxazepam may be longer than that of a single dose of diazepam.

The pharmacokinetic attribute "half-life" becomes clinically significant when benzodiazepines are prescribed in multiple doses over a period of time. When given at frequent, regular intervals, the benzodiazepine blood level builds to a steady state in about five half-lives. Thus, it takes considerably longer to reach steady state with long half-life drugs than short half-life drugs. Once steady state has been reached, it takes five half-lives for drugs to be more than 90% eliminated from the body after drug dosing has been discontinued. Thus, elimination of long half-life benzodiazepines is also considerably slower than that of short half-life drugs. Knowledge of benzodiazepine elimination half-life times is therefore of importance primarily when considering attainment of steady-state blood levels or discontinuance of the medication (Shader and Greenblatt 1977).

The pharmacokinetic characteristics of various benzodiazepines that are available for clinical use in the United States are shown in Table 1.

Development of Tolerance

Long-term use of benzodiazepines raises the possibility of the development of tolerance to the therapeutic effects. Pharmacologically, the development of tolerance to the sedative and psychomotor effects of benzodiazepines is well documented (Aranko et al. 1983; Busto and Sellers 1986; Fabre et al. 1981; File 1981, 1982a, 1982b; Gallager et al. 1984; Greenblatt and Shader 1978; Haefely 1986; Hollister et al. 1981; Lucki et al. 1986), but there are conflicting reports about the development of tolerance to anxiolytic effects of benzodiazepines. Research studies do not report development of tolerance to therapeutic effects (Laughren et al. 1982a; Maletzky and Klotter 1976; Marks 1983; Rickels et al. 1983). In the treatment of patients with panic disorder, researchers have noted a dose reduction over time (Burrows, in press; Sheehan 1987). Some clinicians, however, have observed slight increases in benzodiazepine doses over time (Gordon 1967; Khan et al. 1980; Lin et al. 1989), suggesting the development of mild tolerance to the therapeutic effect (Böning 1985). These dose increases are usually small, and long-term use does not lead to significant dosage increases over time or to high-dose abuse (Balmer et al. 1981; Garvey and Tollefson 1986). However, these clinical observations suggest that there is differential development of tolerance to the different effects of benzodiazepines and allows for the possibility that there may be mild tolerance to antianxiety effect in some patients. The mechanism of tolerance is receptor related and is not due to pharmacokinetic changes (Christensen 1973; Crawley et al. 1982; File 1981, 1982a, 1982b; Gallager et al. 1984; Haigh and Feely 1988), since benzodiazepines do not induce their own metabolism. There is no evidence to suggest that tolerance results from any increased production of endogenous ligands (Lader and File 1987).

3

Patterns of Benzodiazepine Use

BENZODIAZEPINES are among the most widely used drugs in the world. Information regarding their use derives primarily from two sources, surveys of drug prescribing practices and probability-based household surveys of drug use.

Patterns of Benzodiazepine Prescription

One and one-half billion benzodiazepine prescriptions were filled in U.S. drugstores from 1965 to 1985: approximately 1.3 billion for anxiolytics and almost 200 million for hypnotics. Most prescribing of benzodiazepine is by nonpsychiatrists, mainly general practitioners and internists (Woods et al. 1987). In 1965, not long after the first benzodiazepine was released for clinical use, retail pharmacies dispensed 30 million prescriptions for the benzodiazepine anxiolytics. By 1973, this figure had increased to 87 million. Prescription volume remained stable for the next two years, then decreased annually to 55 million prescriptions in 1981. Between 1981 and 1985, the number of anxiolytic prescriptions rose annually, but at a much lower rate of increase than that reported from 1965 to 1973. Data on the number of benzodiazepine anxiolytic prescriptions dispensed in 1985, 1986, and 1987 by retail pharmacies suggest that the annual volume of prescriptions for these medications has leveled off at about 61 million, and is approximately equal to the total number of benzodiazepines dispensed in 1970. Annual number of prescriptions for benzodiazepine hypnotics has increased steadily from 1970 to 1985, but the prescription volume for the entire hypnotic class, including nonbenzodiazepines, has declined sharply in the same period.

In 1965, chlordiazepoxide accounted for 70%, and diazepam accounted for 27% of all medically prescribed benzodiazepines. Prescription volume for both drugs rose over the next five years, but diazepam prescriptions increased more dramatically and represented over half of the market by 1970. By 1975, diazepam's market share had risen to 70%. Both market share and prescription volume for chlordiazepoxide decreased steadily from 1970 to 1985, while diazepam remained the most commonly prescribed benzodiazepine, with a prescription volume more than twice that of its nearest competitor.

The pattern of benzodiazepine prescribing has shifted with time. Since their introduction into medicine, both lorazepam and alprazolam have been increasingly prescribed, with a concomitant decrease in prescriptions for diazepam. By 1984, lorazepam accounted for 15.3% of drugstore prescriptions for benzodiazepine anxiolytics, and alprazolam accounted for 13.2%. By December 1987, alprazolam had overtaken diazepam, so that alprazolam became the most prescribed benzodiazepine of all (Nelson 1987).

National Household Surveys of Benzodiazepine Use

In addition to drug prescription data, several probability-based household surveys of benzodiazepine use among persons in the general national population have been conducted in the United States, as well as in Europe. National household survey data for the United States in 1979 and 1981 showed that approximately 11% of the adult population had taken an anxiolytic one or more times during the previous year. Forty-five percent of the use was occasional (defined as one or two days at a time), and almost all of this use was for a total of 30 days or less. For 80% of all anxiolytic users, the longest period of daily use was less than 4 months, and for 67%, the longest period of use was less than 1 month. However, for 15% of the anxiolytic users (1.65% of the total population), the longest period of daily use was 12 months or longer. (For 5% use was between 4 and 11 months) (Balter et al. 1984; Mellinger et al. 1984a, 1984b). One-third of these long-term users have been taking these medications regularly for over 7 years; two-thirds for over 3 years. Thus, the existing pool of long-term users had been accumulating very slowly over time. For psychiatric patients, as compared with other patients, use rates were higher and chronic administration was more characteristic. Women tended to take benzodiazepines at twice the rate for men. In 10 Western European countries and the United States, past-year prevalence rates ranged from 7.4% (the Netherlands) to as high as 17.6% (Belgium). The proportion of past-year users who had taken these medications daily for 12 months or more varied by country from a high of 33% (Belgium) to a low of 6% (Sweden). Italy, the United States, and Germany at 14% were in the middle range. The 1.5% prevalence rate of long-term use in the general United States population is one-half as much as the 3.0% long-term prevalence use in Great Britain (Balter et al. 1984). European women also took benzodiazepines about twice as often as men.

In the United States long-term users (12 months or longer) could be distinguished from shorter-term users. They were older, had substantial psychological distress (including depression), and had significant somatic health problems, especially cardiovascular disorders and arthritis (Mellinger et al. 1984a, 1984b). Three recent surveys of long-term benzodiazepine prescription in Britain also demonstrated that most long-term benzodiazepine users were elderly, female, and suffered from physical illness and depressive symptoms (Catalan et al. 1988; Nolan and O'Malley 1988; Rodrigo et al. 1988).

The United States household survey data describe the benzodiazepine usage patterns of patients who took the drugs on a regular or an occasional basis, and thus provide baseline data for estimating the potential incidence of dependence on a therapeutic dose of a *medically supervised* benzodiazepine prescription. The 1979 household survey also reported that approximately 3.5% of the total population took benzodiazepines one or more times that were *not prescribed* for them (Mellinger and Balter 1981; Uhlenhuth et al. 1984). These pills were usually borrowed from a friend or spouse. In a later survey, this figure increased to 5% (Miller et al. 1983; Smith and Nacev 1978). Almost all of these people took benzodiazepines for symptom relief rather than recreational purposes, and almost all took the pills only once or twice.

Patterns of Long-Term Benzodiazepine Use and Dependence

Although data on annual volume of benzodiazepine prescribing and household survey studies of prevalence and pattern of use do not suggest either a recent increase in the amount of medication consumed or an increase in the prevalence of use, there is a continuing public perception that benzodiazepine use is too widespread in the United States as well as in European countries.

This divergence between public attitudes and perception versus actual data on the extent and nature of benzodiazepine use has existed since the first comprehensive report of benzodiazepine use by Marks (1978). This early literature survey suggested that benzodiazepines, in fact, were not over used, and that long-term use or dependence was a relatively limited clinical phenomenon. Although numerous articles in the medical literature from 1975 to approximately 1985 supported these conclusions, reports appearing in the nonmedical literature, autobiographical accounts, and consumer advocate groups all warned against the dangers of overprescribing, long-term use, and dependence on benzodiazepines. Within the past several years, there has also been a rapidly increasing concern on the part of patients as well as some clinicians that dependence may develop more readily to the newer short half-life benzodiazepines such as alprazolam, triazolam, and lorazepam, than to the older compounds such as diazepam or chlordiazepoxide.

There appear to be four groups of long-term regular benzodiazepine users. The first are older patients with a high proportion of medical as well as depressive and other psychiatric illnesses. A second group of long-term regular users are patients who have chronic anxiety and dysphoric symptoms, sometimes with associated personality disorders. These patients appear more typically in psychiatric practice. There are no survey data specifically focusing on this second population of patients, and estimates of the number of these patients and their actual benzodiazepine using habits are not available. Clinical experience suggests that these chronically dysphoric patients seek regular psychiatric attention or regular medical attention, and have their benzodiazepine prescriptions continually renewed. They do not increase their dose (Balmer et al. 1981), and experimental data suggest that anxiety per se does not increase the risk of benzodiazepine dependence (De Wit et al. 1986; Winstead et al. 1974). The patients may have greater difficulty discontinuing benzodiazepines than do patients without personality disorders (Golombok et al. 1987; Tyrer et al. 1983). For these two groups of patients, the medically ill, or the chronically dysphoric, who comprise the majority of chronic users, long-term use appears to be a rational medical therapy. However, depending on one's medical opinion, it may be that some of these long-term users (a significant number of people) do not have clear-cut indications for ongoing regular benzodiazepine therapy. Controversy regarding risk versus benefits of long-term benzodiazepine use centers around this very point: those who emphasize the therapeutic benefit for the majority of long-term user patients versus those who emphasize the risks of long-term use without clear medical indication and the development of dependence. One review suggests that the evidence for long-term anxiolytic efficacy of benzodiazepines is not sufficiently compelling to warrant continuous, uninterrupted use for months or years (Rickels and Schweizer 1987). Other authors emphasize the clinical benefit of ongoing benzodiazepine treatment, especially for the medically ill and clinically dysphoric, with little risk of serious toxicity (Marks 1985).

There are two other currently emerging groups of long-term regular benzodiazepine users who deserve attention. These are patients who take benzodiazepines for reasons other than treatment of anxiety or sleep disturbance. Since there are no current survey data regarding these patients, estimates of their numbers or descriptions of their benzodiazepine using practices cannot be definitively made. The largest cohorts of these newly emerging long-term regular benzodiazepine users are patients who have panic disorder with or without agoraphobic symptoms, and who are being treated most typically with alprazolam, often at doses 4 mg/day or higher. (Some patients may take clonazepam or lorazepam, but during the period this report was being prepared, alprazolam was the benzodiazepine that was overwhelmingly favored for the treatment of panic disorder.) Most clinical studies suggest that patients taking alprazolam for this therapeutic purpose do not abuse the medication or escalate their dose. Like the chronically dysphoric or medically ill patient, long-term benzodiazepine treatment of panic may be appropriate for some patients. A second group of newly emerging long-term benzodiazepine users are patients with psychiatric illness such as schizophrenia, who are being treated primarily with nonbenzodiazepine medication, but who are also being given benzodiazepines for treatment of coexisting anxiety, for adjunctive antipsychotic affect, for diminution of extrapyramidal symptoms, or for treatment of tardive dyskinesia. Although these indications for benzodiazepine use are less well established than the "traditional" antianxiety, hypnotic, or antipanic indications, recent clinical experience with schizophrenic patients suggests that long-term benzodiazepine use is not unusual. There seems to be no dose escalation in these patients, but the rationale for long-term benzodiazepine treatment has not been clearly established.

In summary, available data suggest that benzodiazepines are widely used in clinical practice and although there is not an epidemic of use or overuse, prevalence rates in the general population indicate significant use of these compounds. General concerns about the overprescribing and misuse of medications often do not hold up when they are translated into specific research questions and confronted by relevant data. For example, in the United States during the mid- and late 1970s, public concerns about the overprescribing and misuse of antianxiety/sedative medications were intense. Despite the public clamor, when the requisite survey research studies were performed, data indicated that a high proportion (60%) of persons who were legitimate candidates for therapy had not sought or obtained treatment of any kind for their psychological problems. Only 33% of those classified high on symptoms of anxiety *and* depression had been treated with any psychotherapeutic medication (28% treated with an antianxiety/sedative medication) (Balter 1988). Likewise, among persons who met stringent criteria for psychiatric syndromes, the proportion who had been treated with psychotherapeutic medications or psychosocial therapies was surprisingly low. In the case of both major depression and generalized anxiety, the treatment rate was under 40% (Uhlenhuth et al. 1983, 1984, 1988). Only for agoraphobia-panic, a very disabling low-prevalence disorder, did the rate of treatment exceed 40%.

Another way of gauging whether medication is being over-prescribed or misprescribed is to determine whether the patients receiving benzodiazepine treatment merit prescription of these drugs. Are recipients of medications legitimate candidates for therapy? Once again, U.S. survey data indicate that they were. A high proportion of the recipients of antianxiety medications met clinical criteria for psychiatric illness. Sixty-six percent of those patients treated with antianxiety medications suffered from very high psychic distress, had experienced serious life crises, or both (26%). Only 7% scored low on ratings of both psychic distress and life crisis (Balter 1988).

From an epidemiological point of view, therefore, medical treatment with antianxiety/sedative medications does not seem to present any great public health problems. Data even suggest that anxiolytics may actually be underprescribed to anxious patients (Nagy 1987); a substantial majority of persons who reported a high level of psychic distress did not use medically prescribed psychotherapeutic drugs (Mellinger et al. 1974). Furthermore, therapeutic use of benzodiazepines without medical supervision in the general population is rare (Woods et al. 1988). From the clinical and consumer perspective, however, there are problems of overuse, drug dependence, and abuse.

However, since clinical experience and public perception do not necessarily correspond to available survey data, the question of overall benzodiazepine use as well as shifting patterns of prescription must continue to be accurately surveyed and otherwise monitored. The survey data in the United States used for this report were collected prior to the introduction of alprazolam and therefore were conducted at a time when diazepam was still the most widely prescribed benzodiazepine. Since December 1987, alprazolam has become the most widely prescribed benzodiazepine in the United States, and triazolam has become the most widely prescribed benzodiazepine hypnotic. The question of overuse, misuse, dependence, or long-term use of any drug can never be examined during the early months or the first year of widespread prescription, since most patients are still in the early stages of therapeutic drug use. Therefore, if it is true that long-term use and dependence on these newer benzodiazepines is a growing public health concern, even though overall benzodiazepine use is not increasing, then new survey data will be required to demonstrate this phenomenon. The American patient population is neither well served by misguided impressions nor by anachronistic data.

4

Physiological Dependence
on Benzodiazepines

Definitions

Abrupt discontinuance of many drugs will result in the development of signs and symptoms of discontinuance. In daily life, discontinuance symptoms are commonly experienced when nicotine, caffeine, and alcohol are stopped. In medical practice, steroids, anticoagulants, beta-blocking cardiovascular agents, and anti-inflammatory drugs are common examples of drugs that must be tapered in order to avoid discontinuance signs and symptoms (Haefely 1986; Morgan et al. 1973). All psychiatric drugs, if taken for more than a brief period, may produce discontinuance signs and symptoms when abruptly stopped, and these symptoms may be an intensified recurrence of the original signs and symptoms, or may be the mirror image (for example, the opposite of the normal therapeutic effect of the drug). Sudden discontinuance of antidepressant drugs, for example, may produce a severe depression, rebound cholinergic symptoms, or agitation, or it may precipitate a manic state (Charney et al. 1982). Withdrawal dyskinesia is commonly seen after neuroleptics are abruptly stopped, and a recrudescence of manic symptoms has been reported after abrupt lithium termination.

Among other classes of drugs, the sedative-hypnotics and opioids are commonly associated with characteristic discontinuance phenomena. Typically, the common and important signs and symptoms that are produced when these drugs are abruptly stopped are the mirror image of the effect of the drug and are characteristic enough to be denoted by the term *abstinence syndrome*. Thus, discontinuance of a sedating drug will produce arousal: agitation, insomnia, restlessness, and anxiety. Benzodiazepines are sedative-hypnotic drugs and share many of their characteristics, including the development of discontinuance symptoms following abrupt termination.

The presence of a predictable physical abstinence syndrome following abrupt discontinuance of benzodiazepines is evidence of the development of physiological dependence. It was formerly believed that such physiological dependence occurred only when high doses of benzodiazepines were taken, especially over long periods of time. Historically, long-term, high-dose physiological dependence has been called addiction, a term that implies recreational abuse. In recent years, however, it has become apparent that physiological adaptation develops and discontinuance symptoms can appear after regular daily therapeutic dose administration (Lader 1984; Lader and Petursson 1983a), in some cases after only a few days or weeks of administration. Since therapeutic prescribing is clearly not recreational abuse, the term *dependence* is preferred to addiction, and the abstinence syndrome is called a *discontinuance syndrome.*

In this section discontinuance will be described, and distinctions will be drawn between common and uncommon symptoms, as well as between severe and less severe symptoms. Special emphasis will be placed on a description of the most serious discontinuance symptoms—seizures, as well as a description of some of other common discontinuance symptoms.

Description of Discontinuance Symptoms

The benzodiazepine discontinuance syndrome can be divided into three categories of symptoms: rebound, recurrence, and withdrawal (Greenblatt and Shader 1978; Noyes et al. 1988b; Salzman 1984) (Table 2).

Rebound symptoms are a return of the original symptoms for which the benzodiazepine was prescribed, transiently in a more intense form than before treatment. Originally described as rebound insomnia following discontinuance of hypnotic drugs, in-

Table 2.   Symptoms of benzodiazepine discontinuance syndrome

Symptom category	Type of symptoms	Severity compared to original symptoms	Course
Rebound	Same as original	More	Rapid onset and temporary
Recurrence	Same as original	Same	Very gradual onset; does not disappear with time
Withdrawal	New symptoms	Variable	Occurs early or late; lasts 2–4 weeks (occasionally longer)

cluding benzodiazepines (Kales et al. 1978, 1979), it is now recognized that rebound anxiety can occur when antianxiety agents, including benzodiazepines, are abruptly terminated.

If the cause of the original symptoms has not been corrected, then the same pattern and intensity of symptoms may recur after the benzodiazepines have been discontinued. This return of symptoms is called recurrence (or relapse or recrudescence) and is likely when benzodiazepines have been prescribed for only a brief period of time. Unlike rebound symptoms, the original symptoms that recur following discontinuance persist over time and are not more severe. Following chronic benzodiazepine treatment of more than one year duration, recurrent anxiety has been reported in as many as 50%–65% of patients (Golombok et al. 1987; Rickels et al. 1986b). Among panic disorder patients, recurrence may be as high as 95% (Sheehan 1986). There is considerable overlap between the symptoms of recurrence and rebound, and some authors consider many discontinuance symptoms to be recurrence (Greenblatt et al. 1983a, 1983b). Others, however, strongly advocate the distinction between recurrence, which only suggests that the original symptoms have not been adequately treated, and discontinuance symptoms such as rebound, which suggest physiological change induced by the drugs themselves (Ashton 1984; Bixler et al. 1985; Busto et al. 1986b; Lader and Petursson 1983c; Mackinnon and Parker 1982; Rickels et al. 1988a; Tyrer and Seivewright 1984). Clinically, it may be impossible to discriminate between rebound and recurrence, and both discontinuance phenomena may occur together. Thus, a common pattern of discontinuance symptoms is the occurrence of an immediate worsening of symptoms shortly after the patient stops the benzodiazepine (rebound). After a few days the original symptoms (usually anxiety or insomnia) lessen and return to their predrug intensity (or below) and then persist (recurrence).

The term *withdrawal* specifies the development of new signs and symptoms and worsening of preexisting symptoms following drug discontinuance that were not part of the disorder for which the drugs were originally prescribed. Examples of withdrawal symptoms include photophobia, auditory and visual hypersensitivity, tinnitus, and seizures. Withdrawal symptoms define a true *abstinence syndrome* and suggest that there is physiological change as a consequence of the drug administration. Withdrawal symptoms tend to develop together with rebound and recurrence and may persist up to several weeks (occasionally for months). Like the withdrawal symptoms that develop after discontinuance of other sedative-hypnotic drugs, benzodiazepine withdrawal symptoms may be severe,

Table 3. Benzodiazepine anxiolytic discontinuance symptoms

Very frequent[a]	Common but less frequent[b]	Uncommon[c]
Anxiety	Nausea	Psychosis
Insomnia	Coryza	Seizures
Restlessness	Diaphoresis	Persistent tinnitus
Agitation	Lethargy	Confusion
Irritability	Hyperacusis	Paranoid delusions
Muscle tension	Aches and pains	Hallucinations
	Blurred vision	
	Depression	
	Nightmares	
	Hyperreflexia	
	Ataxia	

[a] *Sources:* Abernethy et al. 1981, 1983; Adam et al. 1984; Ashton 1984; Barten 1965; Berlin and Conell 1983; Busto et al. 1986b; Lader 1983a, 1983b, 1984, 1987a; Lader and Petursson 1983a, 1983b, 1983c; Lader et al. 1984; Maletzky and Klotter 1976; Noyes et al. 1988a; Pecknold et al. 1982; Petursson and Lader 1981a, 1981b; Rickels et al. 1988a; Schöpf 1981, 1983; Tyrer et al. 1981; Uhlenhuth et al. 1988; Winokur et al. 1980.

[b] *Sources:* Abernethy et al. 1981; Berlin and Conell 1983; Busto et al. 1986b; Fontaine et al. 1984, 1985; Haefely 1986; Haskell 1975, 1976; Higgitt et al. 1985; Lader 1983a, 1983b, 1984, 1987a, 1987b; Lader and Petursson 1983a, 1983b, 1983c; Maletzky and Klotter 1976; Mellor and Jain 1982; Olajide and Lader 1984; Owen and Tyrer 1983; Pecknold et al. 1982; Petursson and Lader 1981a, 1981b; Schöpf 1983; Shur et al. 1983; Winokur et al. 1980.

[c] *Sources:* Ashton 1984; Barton 1981; Busto et al. 1988; Ferholt and Stone 1970; Floyd and Murphy 1976; Fruensgaard 1976; Mellor and Jain 1982; Preskorn and Denner 1977.

may interfere with normal functioning, and may even be life threatening in rare instances.

There are hundreds of reports in the psychiatric and medical literature of benzodiazepine discontinuance symptoms occurring after therapeutic doses. The symptoms tend to fall into three broad categories: 1) frequent signs and symptoms, 2) those signs and symptoms that occur often but less frequently, and 3) signs and symptoms that are characteristic of the discontinuance syndrome, but occur rarely (Table 3).

Withdrawal Seizures

Of all discontinuance symptoms, seizures present an immediate threat to patient health and safety. Benzodiazepines, like other sedative-hypnotics, have been associated with seizures following abrupt discontinuance, but the incidence of benzodiazepine withdrawal seizures is low. Most seizures occurred when higher than therapeutic doses of the long half-life benzodiazepines, primarily diazepam, were abruptly discontinued (Dysken and Chan 1977; Hollister et al. 1961; Robinson and Sellers 1982; Vyas and Carney 1975). Withdrawal seizures were also experimentally induced in animals withdrawn from diazepam (McNicholas et al. 1983). A withdrawal seizure was also reported following abrupt discontinuance of low-therapeutic doses of diazepam (3 mg/day for 3 months) (DeBard 1979; Rifkin et al. 1976). This rare event, however, may be limited to patients with low seizure thresholds. Discontinuance seizures may be qualitatively different in appearance from usual generalized grand mal seizures. For example, symmetrical myoclonic jerks in the presence of a confused mental status sometimes may be seen.

Reports to the U.S. Food and Drug Administration (FDA) and clinical experience suggest that most withdrawal seizures are usually not associated with long half-life benzodiazepines but more often follow abrupt discontinuance of therapeutic doses as well as high doses of short half-life benzodiazepines (Einarson 1981), especially those that are high in potency (Barton 1981; Breier et al. 1984; de la Fuente et al. 1980; Einarson 1980; Howe 1980; Kahan and Haskett 1984; Levy 1984; Nelson 1987; Noyes et al. 1986; Schneider et al. 1987; Soni et al. 1986; Tien and Gujavarty 1985; Tyrer 1980b). Whether or not the higher frequency of reported discontinuance seizures with these short half-life, high-potency benzodiazepines is due to some intrinsic factor of these particular drugs, or is due to more extensive, higher doses or multiple concomitant medications, or more frequent reporting of seizures, cannot be stated. Even with these short half-life benzodiazepines, however, the risk of seizures appears to be low and to be related to abrupt discontinuation of higher than usually recommended doses that have been taken for extended periods of time.

Typically, most withdrawal seizures occurred within 1 to 3 days of discontinuing the drug (de la Fuente et al. 1980; Einarson 1980, 1981; Howe 1980; Levy 1984; Tien and Gujavarty 1985; Tyrer 1980b). In some cases, however, the seizures have occurred after a week or weeks following discontinuation (Barton 1981; de la Fuente et al. 1980; Kahan and Haskett 1984; Noyes et al. 1986; Robinson and Sellers 1982), depending on the elimination half-life of the drug (discussed below).

Since seizures are uncommon, however, other factors must determine the development of withdrawal seizures in addition to pharmacological properties of the benzodiazepine. Withdrawal seizures are also more common in patients taking multiple drugs or who are dependent on other sedative hypnotics, especially alcohol (Clare 1971; Einarson 1981; Soni et al. 1986), and they may be more common in older patients (Barton 1981; Levy 1984).

Taken together, the following factors predispose patients to the development of withdrawal seizures.

1. *Dose and Duration.* Withdrawal seizures are rare when therapeutic doses of benzodiazepines are taken for periods of weeks or months, and most reports in the literature and to the FDA document seizures that are associated with higher than therapeutic doses of anxiolytic or hypnotic benzodiazepines. In nearly all reports, patients who developed withdrawal seizures had taken benzodiazepines for a long period of time, usually for several years.

2. *Pharmacological properties of the discontinued drug.* Clinical experience and reports to the FDA suggest that withdrawal seizures are more common when the short half-life benzodiazepines have been abruptly discontinued. Clinical experience suggests that seizures may be more common following abrupt discontinuation of the high-potency, short half-life benzodiazepines, but this has not yet been conclusively proven. Seizures may also occur following abrupt discontinuance of long half-life benzodiazepines, but less frequently.

3. *Type of discontinuance.* Withdrawal seizures have usually been reported after abrupt benzodiazepine discontinuance. There are only occasional reports of seizures that have developed during the tapering period.

4. *Multiple drug use.* Many of the reports of withdrawal seizures suggest that the presence of other sedative hypnotic drugs, or alcohol, or other psychotropic drugs that lower seizure threshold, such as neuroleptics and tricyclic antidepressants, increase the risk of developing a benzodiazepine withdrawal seizure.

5. The presence of a treated seizure disorder does not, by itself, increase the risk of withdrawal seizures. However, a latent seizure disorder may be unmasked when benzodiazepines are abruptly discontinued.

Temporal Pattern and Intensity
of Discontinuance Symptoms

The symptoms of discontinuance after abrupt termination of benzodiazepine treatment of generalized anxiety disorder have been observed by clinicians to follow a temporal pattern. Most benzodiazepine discontinuance syndromes usually appear within 3 days after discontinuation, reach a maximum intensity from 3 days to 2 weeks, and usually subside in 4 weeks.

These discontinuance symptoms, their intensity, and their duration depend on the pharmacological properties of the benzodiazepine that has been discontinued. Short half-life drugs are associated with an earlier onset of discontinuance symptoms, and a shorter duration than the symptoms that are produced by long half-life benzodiazepines. Discontinuation of long half-life benzodiazepines, in contrast, may not produce symptoms for days or even a week; the symptoms may be of longer duration because of the slower elimination of the benzodiazepines and its active metabolites. Gradual benzodiazepine discontinuation schedules tend to reduce differences between various half-life benzodiazepines.

If all three components of the benzodiazepine discontinuance syndrome are considered together, then the appearance of certain signs and symptoms may occur in a predictable pattern:

1. Anxiety, insomnia, and restlessness begin with the first several days of discontinuance.
2. Signs and symptoms of confusion, tachycardia, hallucinations, depersonalization, and alterations in consciousness occur primarily in the first 10 days.
3. Some symptoms such as tremor, anorexia, sweating, lethargy, nausea, anxiety, agitation, insomnia, myoclonus, tachycardia, and hypertension tend to appear shortly after benzodiazepine discontinuation and usually disappear after 2 to 3 weeks.
4. Perceptual hyperacusis and photophobia may begin after a few days, but sometimes they are not seen until 3 weeks after discontinuance. (These perceptual experiences are sometimes experienced as a tilting or movement of still objects.)

Although most withdrawal symptoms that result from therapeutic doses of benzodiazepine subside in 1 to 4 weeks, an occasional patient may experience symptoms up to three months after discontinuance. The reasons for this prolonged withdrawal syndrome are not known.

Discontinuance Syndrome from
Benzodiazepine Hypnotics

Clinicians commonly prescribe benzodiazepines in order to initiate and maintain sleep. Thirty-five percent of adults report that they have some insomnia during the course of a year, 17% report "serious insomnia," and 2.6% of the general population use a medically prescribed hypnotic during the course of a year, usually only for a few nights at a time. Only 10% of those with serious insomnia use a hypnotic during the course of a year. Eleven percent of all past year hypnotic users (0.3% of all adults) have used hypnotics regularly for 12 months or more (Mellinger et al. 1985).

Benzodiazepines given to promote sleep may be associated with the development of dependence and signs and symptoms of discontinuance. Like the other sedative hypnotic drugs, dependence and withdrawal may occur even when therapeutic doses have been used. Two syndromes of disturbed sleep are associated with sedative-hypnotic discontinuance. The first is *drug-withdrawal insomnia* (Kales et al. 1974), following abrupt discontinuation of nonbenzodiazepine hypnotics such as the barbiturates, chloral hydrate, or others after long-term, multiple-dose prescription. Drug withdrawal insomnia is considered to be part of a general abstinence syndrome resulting from withdrawal of CNS-depressant drugs at high doses for long periods of time. Symptoms include increased sleep latency (time it takes to fall asleep), disrupted and fragmented sleep, and increased dreaming associated with a REM sleep rebound during the withdrawal period.

A second syndrome has been termed *rebound insomnia.* Rebound insomnia may take various forms, but it is usually characterized by increased sleep latency, increased wake time after sleep onset, and reduced total sleep time compared with pretreatment levels (Gillin et al. 1989). Associated primarily with short half-life benzodiazepine hypnotics taken at therapeutic doses, even for brief periods of time (Kales et al. 1979, 1983a, 1983b), rebound insomnia is considered to be a classical withdrawal phenomenon. Like rebound anxiety, the symptoms of withdrawal are those for which the drug was originally prescribed, only more intense. The transient insomnia typically occurs on the first night and sometimes the second after discontinuance of short half-life hypnotics. Beyond this time period, the likelihood of rebound insomnia appears to be low, although lasting rebound has been reported (Adam et al. 1976). This syndrome does not appear to be related either to age or duration of treatment.

It is clinically significant that rebound insomnia rarely occurs, if ever, with long half-life benzodiazepine hypnotics, such as flurazepam (or other less familiar long-acting benzodiazepine hypnotics such as quazepam) (Kales and Kales 1983; Kales et al. 1982). Like the long half-life benzodiazepine anxiolytics, this may be due to the presence of an active metabolite so that the receptor site is uncovered slowly. Some evidence, however, does suggest that sleep disturbance may occur in some patients during the intermediate period (i.e., nights 4–10) after relatively long-term administration of 30 mg of flurazepam.

The risk of rebound insomnia with the intermediate half-life benzodiazepine hypnotic temazepam is low. No significant rebound insomnia has been observed, even after 33 consecutive nights of treatment, although some subjects have reported a nonsignificant increase in wake time after sleep onset for three withdrawal nights (Mitler et al. 1979). In addition, significantly increased wakefulness has been observed during part of the first withdrawal night following temazepam. Therefore, it is possible that a milder form of rebound insomnia may be associated with temazepam.

Of all the benzodiazepine hypnotics, rebound insomnia has been most regularly observed following use of short half-life compounds (Bixler et al. 1985; Kales and Kales 1983; Kales et al. 1983a, 1983b; Mellinger et al. 1985; Ratna 1981). Rebound insomnia most commonly occurs following discontinuance of the very short half-life benzodiazepine triazolam, but it has also been reported following other short half-life benzodiazepine hypnotics (Kales et al. 1979). The type of insomnia varies among individuals, but the sleep disturbance is generally characterized by reduced total sleep time and efficiency and increased sleep latency and total wake time.

Triazolam rebound insomnia may be partially related to dose. Symptoms have been observed more commonly after treatment with 0.5 mg, rather than with 0.25 mg. Clinical experience suggests that rebound insomnia can occur after a single dose of 0.5 mg (Dement 1986), although it occurs more frequently after multiple doses. Rebound insomnia may develop after less than 1 week of nightly administration (Bixler et al. 1985) and may persist for as long as 2 weeks after discontinuance (Adam et al. 1976). Gradual dose tapering can greatly reduce the intensity of rebound insomnia (Greenblatt et al. 1987a).

Daytime rebound anxiety has been reported by some authors following triazolam discontinuance (Morgan 1982) but not by others (Bliwise et al. 1988).

5

Risk Factors for Clinically Important Physiological Benzodiazepine Dependence

DESPITE THE OBSERVATION that physiological dependence can develop in response to therapeutic doses of benzodiazepines, as indicated by rebound and withdrawal signs and symptoms, not all patients become dependent or develop discontinuance symptoms. In addition to alterations in CNS functioning that are necessary for dependence to develop, many other factors play a role in the etiology of benzodiazepine dependence. Some of these factors are 1) dose and duration of drug use, 2) possible pharmacological differences among the benzodiazepines, and 3) differences among the benzodiazepine users.

High Dose

All sedative-hypnotic drugs, including the benzodiazepines, produce a physiological dependence and discontinuance syndrome in proportion to the amount of drug that has been consumed. The correlation between dose and the severity of the dependence has been established in animal studies (Redmond 1986). Clinically, the higher the dose of benzodiazepine, the more it is likely that the patient will experience symptoms upon drug discontinuance. High-dose dependence has been reported with long half-life benzodiazepines (Abernethy et al. 1981; Allgulander and Borg 1978; Ashton 1984; De Bard 1979; Hollister et al. 1961; Lader 1983a; Ladewig 1984; Laux and Puryear 1984; Mellor and Jain 1982; Pevnick et al. 1978; Preskorn and Denner 1977) and with short half-life drugs as well (Adam et al. 1984; Barton 1981; de la Fuente et al. 1980; Einarson 1980, 1981; Noyes et al. 1985, 1986; Ratna 1981; Selig 1966; Vital-Herne et al. 1985).

There is no minimum "high dose" that predicts the development of dependence without the contribution of other variables such as duration of dosing, type of drug, and factors within the patient. With the introduction of alprazolam (and, to a much lesser extent, lorazepam) as treatments for panic or agoraphobic disorder, higher doses of these benzodiazepines than their usual antianxiety doses are sometimes required for long periods of time to achieve maximum efficacy. The use of these high doses may predispose panic or agoraphobic patients to develop dependence. Recent data from a large 8-week study of patients treated with alprazolam for panic disorder indicate that clinically significant discontinuance symptoms occurred in 35% of patients even after gradual tapering from the high dose (Pecknold et al. 1988). There are no reports indicating the minimum time necessary to develop clinically significant discontinuance symptoms following abrupt withdrawal of high-dose alprazolam or lorazepam treatment of panic disorder, but clinical experience suggests that significant discontinuance symptoms may occur after 4–6 weeks of treatment (see the section on "Patterns of Long-Term Benzodiazepine Use and Dependence" that begins on page 9). Schweizer et al. (1988) observed that after patients with panic disorder had been treated with alprazolam in a daily dosage range from 4 mg to 10 mg for 8 months and were then subjected to a gradual taper discontinuation, over 90% of all patients experienced marked withdrawal symptoms, usually towards the end of the taper period, and 26% of the patients were unable to stay off their benzodiazepine for longer than 1 to 3 days.

Therapeutic Dose

The concept of *therapeutic dose dependence* is common throughout medicine and psychiatry. Patients may become physiologically dependent on many psychiatric and medical drugs that are taken at therapeutic doses, and discontinuance symptoms may occur when these drugs are abruptly stopped. There are numerous reports of physiological dependence in response to therapeutic doses of long half-life benzodiazepines (Abernethy et al. 1981; Agrawal 1978; Allgulander 1978; Ashton 1984; Athinarayanan et al. 1976; Barten 1965; Berlin and Conell 1983; Busto et al. 1986a, 1986b; Covi et al. 1969, 1973; Dietch 1983; Dysken and Chan 1977; Fleischhacker et al. 1986; Floyd and Murphy 1976; Fontaine et al. 1984, 1985; Lader 1983a, 1984; Lader and Petursson 1983b; Laughren et al. 1982b; Laux and Puryear 1984; MacKinnon and Parker 1982; Maletzky and Klotter 1976; Marks 1981, 1983, 1985; Murphy et al. 1984; Owen and Tyrer 1983; Pecknold et al. 1982; Pevnick et al. 1978; Rickels 1981, 1983; Rickels et al. 1980, 1983, 1984, 1986c; Rifkin et al. 1976;

Robinson and Sellers 1982; Schöpf 1981, 1983; Tyrer et al. 1981, 1983; Tyrer and Seivewright 1984; Winokur et al. 1980) as well as in response to therapeutic doses of short half-life benzodiazepines (Adam et al. 1984; Barton 1981; Cohn and Noble 1983; Cohn and Wilcox 1984; Pecknold et al. 1988; Rickels et al. 1986a; Stewart et al. 1980; Tien and Gujavarty 1985; Zipursky et al. 1985).

Duration of Dosing

For clinicians, the most important question concerning the development of tolerance is the amount of time necessary for therapeutic doses to produce clinically meaningful signs and symptoms on discontinuation. In patients who are prescribed benzodiazepine doses within the therapeutic range, duration of treatment is a more important factor for the development of dependence than is the actual dose (MacKinnon and Parker 1982; Rickels et al. 1984). Combining factors of dose and duration, there is a shortened time frame for the development of discontinuance symptoms when higher than usual therapeutic doses are used.

This relationship between dose and duration suggests that if the dose remains within the therapeutic range, then the number of days to produce clinically meaningful dependence and discontinuance symptoms is the critical variable (Himmelhoch 1986). When higher doses are used, the time frame (number of days) to develop dependence and discontinuance symptoms is shortened. Case reports have indicated that dependence on therapeutic doses may occur in some patients after less than 4 weeks of benzodiazepine treatment, as suggested by the appearance of mild discontinuance symptoms (Anonymous 1985; Higgitt et al. 1985). For some short half-life antianxiety benzodiazepines, such as alprazolam, rebound anxiety may be experienced several hours after the last dose. This rebound anxiety is often misinterpreted by the patient as a recurrence of the original anxiety that appears as the drug "wears off."

Rebound insomnia has been reported after only 1 week of therapeutic doses of benzodiazepine hypnotics (Dietch 1983). In most cases, however, rebound anxiety and insomnia are mild and transient. For example, several studies suggest that 4–6 weeks of regular administration of doses in the therapeutic range for treatment of anxiety will produce discontinuance symptoms in some patients (Adam et al. 1984; Barton 1981; Bowden and Fisher 1980; Fontaine et al. 1984; Higgitt et al. 1985; Lader 1987a; Lader and File 1987; Murphy et al. 1984; Pecknold et al. 1982, 1988; Power et al. 1985; Rickels 1987; Rickels and Schweizer 1987), but these rebound symptoms are also usually mild and usually do not interfere with normal functioning (Rickels et al. 1988c). In a small number of people who take short half-life benzodiazepines for 4–6 weeks at therapeutic antianxiety doses, however, the rebound symptoms may be more intense (Rickels et al. 1988c; Wilbur and Kulvik 1983). Nevertheless, most observers have concluded that the occurrence of clinically meaningful symptoms other than mild rebound anxiety and insomnia is low during the first 3–4 months of regular therapeutic dose administration.

After four months of regular, daily therapeutic antianxiety dosing, the development of discontinuance symptoms, including withdrawal and rebound symptoms, increases in likelihood, and the symptoms themselves are more likely to be severe enough to cause additional suffering for the patient (Anonymous 1985; Ayd 1979; Barten 1965; Bowden and Fisher 1980; Breier et al. 1984; Busto et al. 1986a; Covi et al. 1969; Higgitt et al. 1985; Lader 1983b; Lader and Petursson 1983b; Marks 1983; Rickels 1983; Rickels et al. 1983, 1984, 1986b; Tyrer et al. 1981). At this point, rebound anxiety and insomnia are sufficiently severe so that some patients become increasingly reluctant to terminate benzodiazepine use. Percentages of patients reported to be dependent after 6 or more months of continuous, therapeutic-dose benzodiazepine therapy range from as low as 0–40% (Rickels et al. 1983; Tyer et al. 1981) to 82% (Rickels et al. 1986a, 1986b). With such a wide range of clinical reports, accurate estimates of true incidence of clinically meaningful dependence are difficult to make. Double-blind, controlled, prospective studies, however, have confirmed clinical observations that 4–8 months seems to be the critical time period for the development of therapeutic dose dependence (Covi et al. 1973; Rickels and Schweizer 1987; Rickels et al. 1983, 1988).

After 1 year of regular, daily, therapeutic antianxiety dosing of benzodiazepines, the likelihood of dependence and the development of clinically meaningful symptoms upon discontinuance is considerably higher (Winokur et al. 1980). It has been suggested that a large percentage of people who have taken benzodiazepines daily for at least 1 year will experience clinically significant discontinuance symptoms following abrupt withdrawal (Rickels et al. 1986a, 1986b).

Patients who receive benzodiazepines for treatment of panic, anxiety, or agoraphobia symptoms often require higher than usual antianxiety doses to achieve symptom relief and, therefore, are more likely to become dependent and to develop discontinuance symptoms within any given number of days. Furthermore, since patients with panic disorder are likely to take these higher benzodiazepine doses for prolonged periods, their exposure to the benzodiazepine is significantly increased, predisposing them to become medication dependent. This is especially true for the development of withdrawal seizures following benzodiazepine discontinuance (Nelson 1987).

Differences Among Benzodiazepines

Benzodiazepine drugs can be distinguished from each other according to the pharmacologic property of elimination half-life. The quantitative character of discontinuance symptoms is similar for long half-life and short half-life benzodiazepine anxiolytic drugs (Rickels et al. 1986a, 1986b). Similarly, there is no difference in the *incidence* of discontinuance symptoms among the anxiolytic benzodiazepines (Rickels et al. 1986a 1986b), when these medications, given at comparable doses and for comparable periods, are abruptly withdrawn. Discontinuance has been reported for long half-life benzodiazepines (Abernethy et al. 1981; Acuda and Muhangi 1979; Agrawal 1978; Allgulander and Borg 1978; Ayd 1981; Barten 1965; Berlin and Conell 1983; De Bard 1979; Dysken and Chan 1977; Floyd and Murphy 1976; Gordon 1967; Hollister 1977; Hollister et al. 1961; Maletzky and Klotter 1976; Mellor and Jain 1982; Minter and Murray 1978; Murphy et al. 1984; Oswald 1985; Relkin 1966; Rifkin et al. 1976; Robinson and Sellers 1982; Vyas and Carney 1975), as well as for the short half-life drugs (Adam et al. 1976; Barton 1981; Breier et al. 1984; Browne and Hauge 1986; de la Fuente et al. 1980; Einarson 1980, 1981; Hanna 1972; Howe 1980; Kahan and Haskett 1984; Kantor 1986; Levy 1984; Mendelson 1978; Misra 1975; Noyes et al. 1985, 1986; Schneider et al. 1987; Selig 1966; Stewart et al. 1980; Tien and Gujavarty 1985; Tyrer 1980b; Vital-Herne et al. 1985; Voltato et al. 1987; Zipursky et al. 1985). However, the time of onset of discontinuance symptoms is more rapid, and the symptoms are often more severe, when short half-life benzodiazepines are abruptly withdrawn compared with long half-life benzodiazepines. These differences between short and long half-life drugs become less distinct when the drugs are gradually tapered.

Among hypnotic drugs, as already indicated, rebound insomnia occurs primarily after abrupt discontinuation of short half-life drugs, but it may also occur to a lesser extent following abrupt discontinuation of long half-life drugs. Rebound insomnia following triazolam, the benzodiazepine with the shortest half-life, is typically maximal on the first withdrawal night and is usually over by the second or third night. Regardless of which benzodiazepine hypnotic is prescribed, the risk of rebound insomnia is clearly higher following treatment with a higher dose, such as 0.5 mg of triazolam compared with 0.25 mg.

In addition to elimination half-life, benzodiazepines can be distinguished from each other according to their therapeutic potency. Although drug potency in a pharmacological sense encompasses several factors related to drug activity at the receptor site, in clinical practice drug potency usually means that therapeutic effect at a low dose equals higher potency, whereas therapeutic effect requiring a high dose equals lower potency. The potency and the half-life are not related, so that there exist a high-potency, short half-life drug (e.g., triazolam) and a high-potency, long half-life drug (e.g., clonazepam), as well as a low-potency, short half-life drug (e.g., oxazepam) and a low-potency, long half-life drug (e.g., chlordiazepoxide). There are no differences in profile or pattern of discontinuance symptoms between high- and low-potency benzodiazepines, although time course and frequency of seizures, as noted, are different.

Since the introduction of the short half-life, high-potency antianxiety benzodiazepines, however, clinicians have begun increasingly to observe clinically important discontinuance symptoms in some patients taking therapeutic doses. The critical variable for predicting the onset and severity of discontinuance symptoms, therefore, is the drug's elimination half-life (Hollister 1981), although not all authors are in agreement (Böning 1985). Presumably, all short half-life benzodiazepines would be expected to produce similar discontinuance syndromes at comparable doses. Furthermore, there are no research data to suggest that therapeutic potency is related to severity of discontinuance. Anecdotal reports and clinical experience, however, have increasingly noted severe discontinuance with the high-potency, short half-life benzodiazepines alprazolam, lorazepam, and triazolam. Severe discontinuance symptoms have been observed in some patients who have taken alprazolam for anxiety as well in those who take higher doses for panic disorder (Breier et al. 1984; Cohn and Noble 1983; Fyer et al. 1987; Herman et al. 1987; Juergens and Morse 1988; Klein 1986; Noyes et al. 1985, 1986; Vital-Herne et al. 1985; Zipursky et al. 1985). Some patients taking alprazolam experience rebound and withdrawal symptoms of sufficient severity so that they are unable or unwilling to discontinue the drug (Herman et al. 1987). In the United Kingdom, similar concern has been expressed about lorazepam (Tyrer and Murphy 1987). As noted, there also have been suggestions that high-potency, short half-life benzodiazepines have been associated with a higher incidence of seizures following abrupt withdrawal. Severe discontinuance symptoms have also been reported with triazolam (Heritch et al. 1987; Schneider et al. 1987; Tien and Gujavarty 1985). Whether or not these more frequent reports of toxicity or severe discontinuance symptoms are due to unique characteristics of these particular drugs or whether they are a consequence of their status as the most prescribed benzodiazepines cannot be determined at this time. It is also apparent that not all patients suffer from severe drug discontinuance symptoms (Laughren et al. 1982b), even when taking short half-life, high-potency benzodiazepines.

Benzodiazepine Dependence and Patient Type

In addition to factors of dose, duration, and pharmacology that are associated with the development of dependence, some patients may be more likely to become dependent on benzodiazepines because of their treatment patterns: four groups of patients in particular are more likely to receive higher doses or a long duration of treatment, thus increasing their risk of physiological dependence: 1) patients with current or prior dependence on sedative hypnotics, including alcohol and previous benzodiazepines; 2) patients who have chronic illnesses (medical or psychiatric); 3) patients who have chronic dysphoria and/or who have personality disorders (borderline or dependent); and 4) patients with chronic sleep difficulties.

There is abundant evidence suggesting that patients who have been previously dependent on a sedative or hypnotic drug, including benzodiazepines, may be at higher risk for becoming dependent again on these drugs. Similarly, those with prior alcohol dependence may be at higher risk (Busto et al. 1983a, 1983b; Ciraulo et al. 1988a, 1988b). It appears that a history of long-term or high-dose sedative-hypnotic drug use with attendant tolerance and dependence facilitates the redevelopment of tolerance to sedative-hypnotics in the future. While experimental evidence in humans is lacking, this concept is congruent with clinical experience and animal studies, which suggest that previously dependent patients may require higher than usual benzodiazepine doses for therapeutic effect (Aranko et al. 1983; Owen and Tyrer 1983).

A second group of patients who are more likely to become dependent are those whose illness is chronic and who therefore need continual benzodiazepine prescription. Unlike those with prior drug or alcohol dependence, these patients are not more susceptible because of any intrinsic alterations in their physiology. Rather, they are at greater risk to develop dependence because they take benzodiazepines for therapeutic purposes for long periods of time. Chronic medically ill patients tend to be older and tend to have at least one chronic and significant physical disorder, often with pain (King et al. 1988; Mellinger et al. 1984b). They also visit their physicians significantly more often than the general age-matched population, and they also tend to complain of symptoms of both anxiety and depression (Rodrigo et al. 1988). These patients are less often college educated, and they have relatively low incomes. Although long-term users are more likely to have seen a mental health professional, most of these patients are seen in primary care settings. Some of these patients might, in fact, fare better on antidepressant medication or some form of psychosocial intervention and clinical management (Mellinger et al. 1984b). Chronically ill psychiatric patients who may take benzodiazepines daily for long periods of time include those with panic disorder, those with chronic psychotic illness, or those with neuroleptic side effects.

The third group of patients likely to develop benzodiazepine dependence from long-term use are those with chronic dysthymia, dysphoria, and/or personality disorders of the borderline or dependent types (Rickels et al. 1984, 1988b; Tyrer et al. 1983). According to one study, as many as 50% of chronically anxious patients of all ages are not in need of continuous benzodiazepine treatment (Rickels et al. 1984, 1985). For the elderly, who are more sensitive to benzodiazepine effects, long-term treatment may be associated with increased toxicity and dependence (Beers et al. 1988; Lyndon and Russell 1988; Miller and Whitcup 1986; Schneider-Helment 1988; Whitcup and Miller 1987). However, not all patients respond poorly to long term treatment, and for some, long-term treatment may be appropriate therapy. A recent survey of older patients with "tension," for example, indicated that prolonged, low-dose benzodiazepine treatment was safe, helpful, and did not lead to dose escalation, toxicity, or drug abuse (Pinsker and Suljaga-Petchel 1984). Borderline patients, in particular, may be chronically anxious and complain of insomnia, and their symptoms often interfere with their interpersonal functioning, their work, and their self-esteem. Patients with personality disorders commonly depend on sources outside themselves for security, reassurance, and relief of psychic discomfort. Such patients may consume a variety of psychoactive drugs, including benzodiazepines, and they may become dependent or even abuse them. Clinicians commonly are consulted for symptomatic relief, and often benzodiazepines are prescribed on a chronic basis. Although there are no research data regarding this prolonged use of benzodiazepines by dysphoric or personality disorder patients, clinical experience suggests that it is often difficult for these patients to discontinue drug use.

The fourth group of patients who tend to take benzodiazepines on a regular basis are those who use benzodiazepines at bedtime for sleep. Tolerance may develop to the sedative effect of benzodiazepine hypnotics after approximately 2–4 weeks, especially for short half-life benzodiazepines that are administered at therapeutic doses. Some but not all studies indicate that tolerance also develops to long half-life benzodiazepines. It is unclear whether or not these drugs are taken over a long period for their pharmacologic effect or for the *expectation* of their sleep-inducing properties. Patients may also be reluctant to give up these medications because of rebound insomnia. Older patients seem especially reluctant to discontinue these drugs, so it is not unusual to observe a significant number of older residents of nursing homes receiving regular nightly benzodiazepine hypnotics without any clear medical or psychiatric indication for their continued use (Salzman et al. 1989) or evidence that they are still efficacious hypnotics (Linnoila et al. 1980b). This long-term regular use of benzodiazepine hypnotics can produce physiological dependence, with definite discontinuance symptoms.

6

Treatment of Benzodiazepine
Discontinuance Symptoms

S INCE BENZODIAZEPINE DISCONTINUANCE symptoms may cause considerable discomfort, it is not surprising that physicians are confronted with some patients who wish to remain on their medication. A number of strategies have been devised to mitigate or eliminate the discontinuance symptoms. These include 1) gradual dose tapering and 2) substitution of another drug for the benzodiazepine, such as the use of long half-life benzodiazepines (e.g., clonazepam) or the use of nonbenzodiazepines (e.g., propranolol, barbiturates, clonidine, or carbamazepine).

Gradual Benzodiazepine Dose Tapering

Of all the approaches suggested for treating or preventing discontinuance symptoms, gradual tapering is clinically intuitive and has the most clinical support. Several reports provide tapering strategies and document their effectiveness (Fyer et al. 1987; Greenblatt et al. 1987a; Harrison et al. 1984; Marks 1988). In the absence of carefully controlled studies of tapering, the most appropriate approach is simply a slow taper, reducing the first 50% of the daily dose relatively swiftly, the next 25% somewhat slower, and the last 25% very slowly. This slow taper does not guarantee that patients will not experience bothersome withdrawal symptoms, but tapering should prevent the occurrence of psychoses or convulsions. Tapering is particularly important when short half-life, high-potency benzodiazepines such as triazolam and alprazolam are being discontinued (Fyer et al. 1987). Recent clinical experience has suggested (but not proved) that some patients have more difficulty discontinuing these two drugs than other benzodiazepines. For these patients, tapering schedules may have to be prolonged with a very gradual stepwise dose reduction that requires tiny decrements in daily dose. When high doses of alprazolam have been used for the treatment of panic disorder, there is usually little problem in rapidly reducing the dose to a low antianxiety level (e.g., 1–2 mg/day), but further dosage reductions may have to be exceedingly small and gradually instituted, perhaps over weeks or even longer (Fyer et al. 1987).

Drug Substitutes

Long half-life benzodiazepines. Since discontinuance symptoms tend to be more severe with short half-life drugs, clinicians have substituted benzodiazepines with long half-lives and then tapered these drugs slowly. (This strategy has been borrowed from the usual barbiturate tapering procedure in which a long half-life barbiturate is substituted for a shorter half-life drug.) There are, as yet, no research data available to suggest that this substitution of long half-life benzodiazepines is consistently or predictably useful in diminishing or eliminating discontinuance symptoms, and there are no data to suggest the superiority of any particular long half-life benzodiazepine. Use of a loading dose of diazepam (40% of daily consumption), followed by daily tapering by 10% has been reported (Harrison et al. 1984). Although this is a promising clinical approach, substitution of the high-potency, long half-life benzodiazepine (clonazepam) recently has been recommended. Limited clinical experience suggests that substitution of clonazepam, for example, is helpful for some patients who had been unable to discontinue alprazolam (Albeck 1987; Patterson 1988). Clonazepam, however, is a highly potent and often sedating benzodiazepine, so that sedation and incoordination may be sometimes severe during the substitution period. When any long half-life drug is substituted, higher than usual comparable doses may be necessary to suppress the discontinuance symptoms. Furthermore, discontinuance symptoms may still occur even when the long half-life benzodiazepine has been substituted for a short half-life benzodiazepine (Schneider et al. 1987).

Propranolol. Since many of the benzodiazepine discontinuance symptoms suggest autonomic hyperactivity, the use of a beta-blocking drug, such as propranolol, has been recommended (Abernethy et al. 1981; Tyrer et al. 1981). These drugs diminish agitation, muscle twitching, cardiovascular stimulation, diaphoresis, headache, and peripheral symptoms of increased anxiety. The doses necessary for therapeutic effect are variable, and the effects are not predictable or consistent. Side effects, including bradycardia, hypotension, and depression, are not prominent.

Table 4.   Phenobarbital withdrawal conversion doses for
benzodiazepines

Benzodiazepine (generic name)	Dose (mg)	Phenobarbital withdrawal conversion (mg)
Alprazolam	1	30
Chlordiazepoxide	25	30
Clonazepam	4	30
Clorazepate	15	30
Diazepam	10	30
Flurazepam	15	30
Halazepam	40	30
Lorazepam	1	15
Oxazepam	10	30
Prazepam	10	30
Temazepam	15	30

Source. Adapted from Smith and Wesson 1985; Marks 1988.

Clonidine.   The rationale for clonidine treatment of benzodiazepine discontinuance is the same as for propranolol. Clonidine
reduces norepinephrine activity and has been found useful in the
treatment of discontinuance symptoms seen with nicotine, as well
as with opiates. Clinical experience is sparse, and no research studies
are available to guide the clinician (Fyer et al. 1988; Keshavian and
Crammer 1985).

Carbamazepine.   Carbamazepine has been suggested as a possible treatment for benzodiazepine discontinuance seizures. The
drug may also be useful for quieting the CNS hyperarousal that may
follow the abrupt uncovering of inhibitory GABA receptor sites
when benzodiazepines are stopped. Clinical experience with carbamazepine is gradually increasing (Klein 1986; Ries et al. 1989).

Buspirone.   Substitution of buspirone for benzodiazepines
does not prevent or treat the development of benzodiazepine discontinuance symptoms (Jerkovich and Preskorn 1987; Schweizer
and Rickels 1986).

Barbiturates.   The substitution of intermediate or long half-life
barbiturates to attenuate benzodiazepine discontinuance symptoms
has not been widely publicized, but this may be an effective technique for some patients, especially for those with mixed benzo-
diazepine/alcohol dependence. An approximate dose of phenobarbital equivalent to the amount of benzodiazepine is calculated

according to Table 4 (Smith and Wesson 1985). The patient is hospitalized on an inpatient unit and is begun on this phenobarbital dose; benzodiazepines are stopped. The upper daily dose limit is 500 mg/day in three divided doses. If oversedation, unsteady gait, or slurred speech occur, the next dose is withheld. After stabilizing the patient for two days at this calculated dose of phenobarbital, the daily phenobarbital dose is reduced by 30 mg/day.

7

Mechanism of Benzodiazepine
Dependence and Tolerance

THE MECHANISM of benzodiazepine activity at the receptor site is
most likely a major determinant of dependence and withdrawal. As noted in Chapter 2, benzodiazepines bind to the benzodiazepine-GABA receptor complex, enhancing the activity of GABA
to hyperpolarize (decrease excitability of) neurons, thus increasing
CNS inhibitory tone (Paul 1987). Acute behavioral effects are related to the extent of receptor occupancy (Greenblatt et al. 1987b).
Chronic benzodiazepine treatment leads to a GABA down regulation (Cowen and Nutt 1982; Crawley et al. 1982; Gallager and
Lakoski 1984; Greenblatt and Shader 1978; Miller et al. 1988;
Rosenberg and Chiu 1979, 1981, 1982; Rosenberg et al. 1983).
Abrupt dissociation of ("uncovering") benzodiazepines from their
receptors following drug discontinuation may lead to an acute
reduction in GABA (Cowen and Nutt 1982). This, in turn, leads to
a more excitable (less inhibited) CNS, which may be reflected in an
increase in irritability, hyperacusis, myoclonus, seizures, etc. The
loss of GABAergic inhibitory tone following benzodiazepine withdrawal may be likely to be correlated with or even cause the phenomenon of rebound anxiety. A recent report suggests that low
doses and low blood levels of alprazolam and triazolam upregulate
the benzodiazepine receptor (increase receptor number), possibly
explaining interdose rebound symptoms as well as the development
of rebound when the drugs are being tapered (Miller et al. 1987a).

When given regularly over a period of time, benzodiazepine
pharmacokinetics determine the development of discontinuance
symptoms. Abrupt discontinuation of treatment following multiple
dosage is followed by disappearance of the drug from blood, brain,
and receptor site at a rate determined by the drug's elimination
half-life, volume of distribution, and clearance. The time of onset
(and, in part, the intensity) of benzodiazepine discontinuation
syndromes relative to the time of termination of treatment is largely
determined by the drug's elimination half-life (Busto and Sellers

1986). Abrupt discontinuation of short half-life benzodiazepines leads to rapid drug removal from blood and brain, rapid uncovering of the receptor site, and relatively rapid onset of post-drug discontinuance syndromes. In contrast, long half-life derivatives leave the blood and brain slowly after drug discontinuation, "uncover" or dissociate from the receptor correspondingly slowly, and are associated with discontinuance syndromes of slower onset and reduced intensity (Lukas and Griffiths 1982). Because severity of symptoms is related to its half-life, short half-life benzodiazepines given for anxiety are frequently implicated in intense discontinuance syndromes. Daytime rebound anxiety and panic ("clock watching") is associated with falling blood and brain drug levels in between doses of short half-life drugs. Long half-life drugs (chlordiazepoxide, diazepam, desmethyl diazepam, flurazepam) apparently have the lowest likelihood of severe and rapid-onset post-treatment syndromes. With very short half-life drugs such as triazolam, rebound symptomatology has actually been described during the period of drug ingestion, especially when it is given nightly (Morgan and Oswald 1982). This rebound insomnia, occurring during the terminal one-third of the night, is presumably caused by a rapid decline in plasma and brain drug concentrations occurring 4 to 10 hours after dosage. Daytime anxiety has also been attributed to short half-life hypnotics, presumably via a similar mechanism.

It seems, therefore, that both pharmacokinetic and pharmacodynamic factors are associated with both the onset as well as the intensity of therapeutic dose discontinuance symptoms. Short half-life benzodiazepines may be expected to produce an earlier onset of withdrawal symptoms than do longer half-life drugs. Whether or not the severity of these symptoms may also correlate with the therapeutic potency in addition to the kinetics of the compound has yet to be determined.

8

Benzodiazepine Toxicity

General Side Effects

Benzodiazepine drugs produce a spectrum of side effects. The most common of these are drowsiness and sedation. Most patients will experience sedation of varying degrees of severity at the beginning of treatment (Greenblatt et al. 1983a, 1983b). Since tolerance develops to the sedation, this side effect is usually transitory. The degree of sedation depends on the dose, the susceptibility of the benzodiazepine user, and on the pharmacological characteristics of the specific drug. The sedating side effects of benzodiazepines are enhanced by other CNS sedatives; benzodiazepines themselves may augment the sedating effects of other drugs and alcohol. Older patients are more susceptible to benzodiazepine sedation.

Benzodiazepines also commonly cause ataxia, dysarthria, incoordination, diplopia, vertigo, and dizziness (Greenblatt and Shader 1974a, 1974b; Greenblatt et al. 1983a, 1983b). These side effects are related to dose and to individual susceptibility. Older patients are also more susceptible to falls (Granek et al. 1987; Ray et al. 1987; Tinetti et al. 1988).

Unwanted changes in affect associated with benzodiazepine use have been reported, although not with high frequency. These include 1) hostility and 2) depression. Hostility has been noted in some patients who received benzodiazepines, especially under condition of frustration (Kochansky et al. 1975; Salzman et al. 1974, 1975). There is controversy regarding the clinical significance of these observations. One group considers dyscontrol an important effect of benzodiazepines in borderline patients (Gardner and Cowdry 1985), whereas another believes the appearance of hostility to be relatively infrequent and, in most cases, clinically unimportant (Dietch and Jennings 1988). Benzodiazepines have also been reported to cause or to exacerbate symptoms of depression. This, too, is not a frequent side effect, although the depressive symptoms may be potentially serious (Greenblatt and Shader 1974a).

Benzodiazepines have been reported to cause fetal abnormalities. In case reports, diazepam has been associated with an increased rate of oral clefts, dysmorphism, and CNS dysfunction after in utero exposure (Laegreid et al. 1987), although animal studies have shown malformations (Gill et al. 1981). However, some of the mothers described in these reports may also have been taking other licit and illicit drugs, and prospective studies have failed to confirm these case reports. Therefore, reliable data suggest that there is no increased risk of congenital malformations in children who have been exposed only to benzodiazepines during gestation (Cohen et al. 1989). However, benzodiazepine dependence may develop: neonatal withdrawal has been reported in twins born to a mother who was taking therapeutic doses of chlordiazepoxide and diazepam (Athinarayanan et al. 1976; Mazzi 1977; Rementeria and Bhatt 1977). Serious toxic reaction to benzodiazepines have been observed in children (Pfefferbaum et al. 1987).

Benzodiazepines interact with other medications, sometimes with hazardous results. The most common and most serious interaction is with alcohol and with other sedative hypnotics, the combination enhancing CNS sedation. Benzodiazepines also augment the euphoriant effect of opiates. Cimetidine impairs the metabolism of benzodiazepines, but this interaction is not of clinical importance. Other interactions that are of less clinical significance include delay in oral absorption of benzodiazepines when given with antacids and inhibition of biotransformation of some benzodiazepines by disulfiram and oral contraceptives.

Effects on Memory

Benzodiazepines may impair memory function in two distinct ways. First, they may cause an acute amnesia for a brief period of time following high-dose intravenous administration of the drug. Second, and more insidious, is an impairment of recall that occurs during chronic benzodiazepine administration.

There are various theories of memory function that compete for research attention. The theory that is most commonly applied to explain benzodiazepine memory impairment divides memory into several components (Lister 1985; Nicholson and Spencer 1982; Romney and Angus 1984; Roth et al. 1984):

1. *Acquisition:* Information enters via the sensory route.
2. *Retention (short-term memory):* The information is of interest and draws attention.

3. *Consolidation:* Information of interest is transferred to long-term memory.
4. *Retrieval:* This is consolidation in reverse, the obtaining of a memory from long-term storage.

Numerous research studies indicate that benzodiazepines impair memory at the consolidation phase, without impairing sensory intake or retention (Angus and Romney 1984). Thus, a person who has taken a benzodiazepine will be able to remember something that has just been told to them. However, because consolidation is impaired, a person who has taken a benzodiazepine will have trouble remembering something told to them after a period of time. This delayed recall is typical of the effect of benzodiazepines and has been well documented (Angus and Romney 1984; Brown et al. 1978, 1982; Dundee and Pandit 1972; Ghoneim and Mewaldt 1977; Ghoneim et al. 1975, 1981; Grove-White and Kelman 1971; Hartley et al. 1982; Healey et al. 1983; Hinrichs et al. 1982, 1984; Jones et al. 1979; Lister and File 1984; Lucki and Rickels 1986; Lucki et al. 1986, 1987; Mac et al. 1985; Nicholson and Spencer 1982; Petersen 1976; Petersen and Ghoneim 1980; Roehrs et al. 1983, 1984b; Scharf et al. 1983, 1984).

The second type of memory loss is termed *anterograde amnesia* (memory loss after the drug has been taken). It commonly follows high-dose acute intravenous administration (Brown et al. 1978, 1982; Clark et al. 1979; Clarke et al. 1970; Desjardins and Beaver 1982; Dundee and Haslett 1970; Frith et al. 1984; Heisterkamp and Cohen 1975; Long and Eltringham 1977; Pagano et al. 1978; Pandit et al. 1976) and is utilized in benzodiazepine presurgical anesthesia (Brown and Dundee 1968; Dundee and Haslett 1970; McClish 1966; Morgan 1969; Pearce 1974; Poswillo 1967; Stovner and Endresen 1965). However, it has also been reported with increasing frequency when therapeutic oral doses of short half-life, high-potency benzodiazepines (such as triazolam) are taken, especially if taken with alcohol (Bixler et al. 1979; Roehrs et al. 1984a, 1984b; Roth et al. 1980, 1984; Scarone et al. 1981; Shader and Greenblatt 1983; Shader et al. 1986; Spinweber and Johnson 1982). Impairment of memory after oral administration of therapeutic doses of benzodiazepines has typically been tested after a single dose in normal volunteers as well as anxious subjects. The most common deficit is impaired acquisition of new material after a delay in time (Block and Berchou 1984; Desjardins and Beaver 1982; Desjardins et al. 1982; Liljequist et al. 1979; Photiades et al. 1975; Shader and Greenblatt 1983). This drug-induced memory impairment is not associated with the degree of psychomotor impairment and sedation (Roache and Griffiths

1985). Benzodiazepines have no effect on the recall of information that has been learned before the drug was taken (Petersen 1976, Petersen and Ghoneim 1980).

As with other measures of psychologic and psychomotor function, the elderly are more sensitive to the acute memory impairment produced by benzodiazepines (Bonnet and Kramer 1981; Foy et al. 1986; Pomara et al. 1985). The nature of this increased sensitivity is in part due to loss of baseline functional capacity and resiliency to resist the impairing effects of benzodiazepines (Nikaido et al. 1987; Nikaido et al., in press).

There are only a few studies of the long-term effect of therapeutic doses of benzodiazepines on memory, some suggesting impairment (Petursson and Lader 1982). Recent data suggest that when chronic therapeutic doses of benzodiazepines are discontinued, middle-aged and elderly patients subjectively report improved memory function, and objective memory testing shows measurable improvement (Golombok et al. 1988; Salzman et al. 1989).

The effects of benzodiazepines on memory function cannot be briefly summarized. There are differences among the various compounds in their effect on memory, suggesting that high-potency drugs that are also characterized by a short half-life are more likely to impair memory after a single dose (Scharf et al. 1983). Recent studies suggest that therapeutic doses of high-potency, short half-life benzodiazepines impair memory more than comparable therapeutic doses of the low-potency, short half-life drug oxazepam (Curran et al. 1987; Scharf et al. 1987).

Memory impairment also depends on the dose and on the route of administration, with higher doses and intravenous administration causing the greatest impairment. Differences in benzodiazepine users also affects memory. Older patients, and those with a prior history of sedative hypnotic use, were more likely to report memory impairment. Lastly, duration of treatment is a significant factor. Long-term chronic dosing that reduces anxiety may actually improve memory function. In older subjects, however, there may be an insidious, gradual decrement in memory function even at constant doses. Clinicians are also becoming aware that acute anterograde amnesia sometimes follows a single therapeutic dose of the short half-life hypnotic triazolam as well as higher doses of the antianxiety drug lorazepam. The amnestic effects of benzodiazepines may be enhanced by concomitant alcohol ingestion.

Psychomotor Performance

Numerous clinical and experimental studies have documented benzodiazepine-induced impairment of cognitive and neuromotor functioning, primarily in normal experimental subjects, after both acute and chronic dosing regimens (Hindmarch and Gudgeon 1980; Johnson and Chernik 1982; Kleinknecht and Donaldson 1975; Matilla 1984; McLeod et al. 1988; Wittenborn 1979). Psychomotor speed, coordination-ataxia, and sustained attention are examples of tests that respond sensitively to a spectrum of benzodiazepines (Ellinwood and Nikaido 1987), whereas the less sensitive tests involve well-learned capabilities or tasks that are not timed (Johnson and Chernik 1982; Wittenborn 1979).

Benzodiazepines may also improve laboratory performance measures (Lucki et al. 1986) as well as compromising performance. Since psychomotor test performance may be impaired by anxiety, performance may improve when anxiety is reduced by benzodiazepines. Improvement in test performance from this antianxiety effect versus performance impairment from benzodiazepine toxicity is related to dose and subject factors such as age. Toxicity is more likely in older subjects and at higher than usual therapeutic doses.

The effects of long-term administration of benzodiazepines on psychomotor performance are not consistent, vary from study to study, and sometimes are in conflict with each other. For some tests, performance is impaired, and for other tests, performance is not affected. For example, no effects of repeated doses in normal research subjects have been reported for critical flicker fusion, tapping, digit-symbol substitution, choice reaction time, tracking, and arithmetic (Aranko et al. 1985; Bornstein et al. 1985; Borrow and Idzikowski 1979; Church and Johnson 1979; Dimascio and Barrett 1965; Hindmarch 1979a, 1979b; Johanson and Schuster 1986; Lader et al. 1980; Lawton and Cahn 1963; Liljequist et al. 1978; Linnoila and Hakkinen 1974; Linnoila et al. 1977; Mattila 1984; Mendelson et al. 1982; Moskowitz and Smiley 1982; Palva and Linnoila 1978; Palva et al. 1979; Saario 1977; Saario et al. 1976; Salkind and Silverstone 1975; Subhan et al. 1986; Tedeschi et al. 1985). Results of similar tests in anxious patients have also produced inconsistent results with single as well as with repeated doses (Bond et al. 1974; Dimascio and Barrett 1965; Dimascio et al. 1969; Doongaji et al. 1978; Hindmarch 1979a; Linnoila et al. 1980a, 1980b; Malpas et al. 1974; Oblowitz and Robins 1983; Pishkin et al. 1978; Saario 1977; Saario and Linnoila 1976; Saario et al. 1976; Salkind et al. 1979; Tansella et al. 1979).

Several acute dosing studies have reported increased sensitivity to benzodiazepine-induced psychomotor impairments in the elderly as compared to younger subjects (Cook et al. 1983), but these effects may vary among older persons (Morgan 1982; Nikaido et al. 1987; Pomara et al. 1984). Even when studies did not control for severity of concurrent illness or the presence of other medications (e.g., Giles et al. 1978; Reidenberg et al. 1978), there is clear evidence that the elderly are impaired at lower plasma thresholds than are the young (Crooks 1983; Nikaido et al. 1987; Pomara et al. 1985). Clinical observations suggest that stable therapeutic doses of benzodiazepines given regularly to elderly patients may gradually increase psychomotor and cognitive impairment in some patients, and this effect may be most pronounced with long half-life medications (Salzman 1984; Salzman et al. 1983).

Although benzodiazepines produce performance decrements on virtually all tests in single as well as with repeated doses (Carskadon et al. 1982; Cook et al. 1983; Linnoila and Viukari 1976; Mead and Castleden 1982; Morgan 1982; Pomara et al. 1984, 1985) as indicated by diminished function on a large variety of performance measures (Johnson and Chernik 1982; Wittenborn 1980), these impairments are of clinical significance only when they indicate a decreased ability to function in nonresearch laboratory settings. It is difficult to devise experiments to provide the appropriate correlations between laboratory performance and function outside the experimental setting (Landauer 1978, 1981).

However, one of the most important functions outside of the research laboratory that may be compromised by benzodiazepines is the operation of complicated equipment during extended situations that require vigilance. A common example is driving an automobile. Efforts to assess the effects of benzodiazepines on actual driving capabilities include an objective measure of deviations in tracking from the center of the road lane on a highway (O'Hanlon et al. 1982) and ratings of performance on specific car handling tasks, including parking, turning, and braking (Hindmarch and Gudgeon 1980). In addition, a few tests have found a high correlation between accident rates among drivers and their performance on laboratory tests of divided attention decision making, eye tracking, hand-eye coordination, reaction time, and information overload tasks (Hakkinen 1976; McNair 1973; Palva and Linnoila 1978; Palva et al. 1979).

Numerous studies of benzodiazepine effects on actual driving skills have also been performed (Betts and Birtle 1982; Betts et al. 1972; De Gier et al. 1981; Hindmarch and Gudgeon 1980; Hindmarch and Subhan 1983; Hindmarch et al. 1977; Kielholz et al. 1972;

Linnoila and Hakkinen 1974; Linnoila and Mattila 1973; Linnoila et al. 1973; Moskowitz and Smiley 1982; O'Hanlon et al. 1982; Smiley and Moskowitz 1986; Wetherell 1979; Willumeit et al. 1984a, 1984b). These studies have demonstrated that benzodiazepines may impair specific driving skills such as the ability to regulate speed, lane position, passing, and parking, as well as performance in slalom runs, but such effects are not consistent from person to person and may depend on dose and the time of drug administration. Studies of intoxicated drivers (Finkle et al. 1968; Garriott and Latman 1976; Holmgren et al. 1985; Missen et al. 1978a; Neuteboom and Zweipfenning 1984; Peel et al. 1984; Valentour et al. 1980; White et al. 1981; Wilson 1985) as well as drivers in fatal and nonfatal automobile accidents (Bastos and Galante 1976; Berg et al. 1971; Blackburn and Woodhouse 1977; Bo et al. 1975; Cimbura et al. 1982; Fisher 1973; Garriott et al. 1977, 1986; Honkanen et al. 1980; Jick et al. 1981; Krantz and Wannerberg 1981; Missen et al. 1978a, 1978b; Skegg et al. 1979; Terhune and Fell 1982; Vine and Watson 1983; Williams et al. 1986; Woodhouse 1975) suggest that blood levels of benzodiazepines are not higher in drivers who have been involved in automobile accidents. Thus, although benzodiazepines may cause some psychomotor impairment that would suggest an increased risk for operating a car, such impairment is not consistent or predictable, nor are there any data to indicate that benzodiazepine use causes automobile accidents. Benzodiazepines probably impair driving skills most in older persons and in those who have not previously taken such drugs. Repeated, regular *therapeutic doses* of benzodiazepines do not impair automobile driving skills in most people.

The effects of benzodiazepines combined with alcohol are similarly inconsistent. In no case does the combination improve performance. Alcohol and benzodiazepines usually compromise psychomotor performance, and sometimes this impairment is greater than the effect of either of the drugs given alone, especially at higher doses (Erwin et al. 1986; Kleinknecht and Donaldson 1975; Mattila 1984; Seppala et al. 1982). Experimental evidence has confirmed that therapeutic doses of benzodiazepines can act additively with even low blood alcohol levels to produce significant impairment of driving skills (Starmer and Bird 1984). This experimental evidence is confirmed by observations of drivers who had low blood alcohol levels, but who appeared intoxicated and were shown to have therapeutic blood levels of benzodiazepines (Garriott and Latman 1976; Valentour et al. 1980; Wilson 1985).

The benzodiazepines have also been shown to induce ataxia in healthy young and elderly subjects following acute dosing (Ghoneim et al. 1984; Nikaido et al. 1987). Postural unsteadiness may be a special problem in the elderly population since the frequency of falls increases with age (Lipsitz 1988). Although the relationship between the benzodiazepines and falls is unclear at this time, there is convincing evidence that drugs may be an important contributing factor in the occurrence of falls in the elderly (Kramer and Schoen 1984; Macdonald 1985; Ray et al. 1987).

Three studies comprising a small number of patients who had taken benzodiazepines for long periods have noted increased ventricular brain ratios (Lader et al. 1984; Schmauss and Krieg 1987; Uhde and Kellner 1987). These observations have not been confirmed by others (Perera et al. 1987a; Poser et al. 1983; Rickels 1985). The diagnosis of the patients was not similar across the studies, and the patients had other comorbid illnesses as well as multiple drug and alcohol use. Therefore, at this time the interpretation of these preliminary observations do not suggest that the effects of benzodiazepines or benzodiazepine withdrawal produce permanent structural or functional brain damage.

9

Abuse Liability of Benzodiazepines

THE TERMS "misuse" and "abuse" of benzodiazepines are applied to any taking of benzodiazepines that is not medically supervised. It includes the use by individuals who obtain benzodiazepines from nonmedical sources such as family or friends, and who occasionally take these compounds for therapeutic symptom relief (usually anxiety or insomnia), but also patients who use these drugs within the illicit drug culture and take large doses of benzodiazepines recreationally for the purpose of "getting high." The first category may be called unsupervised therapeutic dose misuse, and the latter a true drug abuse which may result in harm to the individual or the individual's social environment.

Unsupervised Use of Benzodiazepines

Clinical observations suggest that there is a significant number of people who keep benzodiazepines available for use, but who rarely take the drugs (Salzman 1984). It would be difficult to consider their occasional self-medication as true therapeutic drug misuse, although it is not strictly under medical supervision.

A more serious form of therapeutic dose misuse occurs in patients who, having had a benzodiazepine once prescribed, continue to take the same therapeutic dose on a regular basis for symptom relief, but without medical supervision. As noted, concern has been expressed over this long-term nonmedically supervised benzodiazepine use, both in the lay literature as well as by psychiatrists. Typically, the person obtains additional medication from different physicians who are not aware of prior prescriptions, or obtains further benzodiazepines from nonmedical sources such as family or friends. In the United States, surveys have determined that the prevalence of unsupervised therapeutic-dose benzodiazepine use for symptom relief rather than for recreational purposes ranges from 2% (Mellinger and Balter 1983) to 5% (Miller et al. 1983; Smith and Nacev 1978) of adults.

A small percentage of patients self-medicate with higher than usual therapeutic doses of benzodiazepines for relief of anxiety, insomnia, or panic. This form of misuse, although unusual, has led to the public health concern that therapeutic doses of benzodiazepines, if continued over time, will gradually escalate to higher and more toxic doses (Busto et al. 1986a; Perera et al. 1987b). Most chronic benzodiazepine users, however, do not escalate their original dose, even after many years.

Several possible explanations for higher than therapeutic dose misuse are possible. If the severity of symptoms increases or if the drug loses its initial effectiveness, some patients may increase their dose in order to maintain therapeutic effect. For example, clinical observations suggest that some patients, particularly those receiving benzodiazepines for panic disorder, may gradually increase their dose in order to maintain therapeutic effect. Subjective distress also may not always be relieved by standard therapeutic doses, and the need for higher than typical therapeutic doses may occur in patients with histories of prior benzodiazepine dependence, or use of sedative/hypnotics or alcohol, indicating either physiological tolerance or an increased psychological need (Ciraulo et al. 1988a, 1988b; Perera et al. 1987b; Woods et al. 1987).

Chronically dysphoric psychiatric patients with dependent personality character structures may also be more likely to exceed original therapeutic dose ranges. Such patients have been characterized as middle-aged women with long histories of psychiatric and somatic illness and a frequent past history of suicide attempt. The dosage used by such women is nearly five times higher than the usual therapeutic benzodiazepine dose, and analgesics and alcohol are also frequently used together with the benzodiazepine (Allgulander 1978). It is difficult to determine the frequency with which psychiatrists or other physicians contribute to such high-dose benzodiazepine use by this group of individuals.

Abuse of Benzodiazepines

A drug has the potential for recreational abuse only if its effects reinforce its own administration (Woods et al. 1987). Benzodiazepines have been taken for recreational purposes, often in high doses, in addition to their traditional therapeutic use for symptomatic relief. However, research with primates as well as with humans (De Wit et al. 1984a, 1984b, 1985; Griffiths and Ator 1981; Griffiths and Roache 1985; Griffiths and Sannerud 1987; Griffiths et al. 1979, 1980, 1981, 1985; Johanson and Uhlenhuth 1980; Ladewig 1984; Orzack et al. 1986; Woods 1982) suggests that the reinforcing effects of benzodiazepines are considerably weaker than those of other drugs of abuse such as other sedative hypnotics, stimulants, and opiates, but the reinforcing effects are stronger than those of drugs recognized as having little abuse potential, such as chlorpromazine.

There is a growing body of data suggesting that there are meaningful differences among the benzodiazepines with respect to their seductiveness as drugs of abuse among the drug-abusing population. These differences are suggested by the results of the following studies:

1. experimental studies of subjective effects and drug self-administration in subjects with histories of drug abuse (Griffiths and Roache 1985);
2. questionnaire or interview studies with drug abusers (Iguchi et al. 1989; Wolf et al. 1989; Woody et al. 1975a);
3. clinical judgment of medical professionals working in drug abuse treatment contexts (Bliding 1978; Griffiths and Wolf 1989; O'Brien and Woody 1986); and
4. epidemiological data on illicit traffic (Bergman and Griffiths 1986; Griffiths et al. 1984).

Taken together, these data suggest that diazepam, in particular, is more reinforcing and has greater abuse potential than do many other benzodiazepines, whereas oxazepam, halazepam, and possibly chlordiazepoxide are weakly reinforcing and may therefore have particularly little abuse potential. Recent clinical observations suggest that alprazolam and, to a lesser extent, lorazepam reinforce their own use and, therefore, like diazepam, have a higher abuse potential than do other benzodiazepines (Perera et al. 1987b; Schmauss et al. 1988). Both diazepam and alprazolam are often purchased illegally on the street. The original source of these medications is thought to be from diversion of legally, although inappropriately, obtained medical prescription (DuPont 1986, 1988). In Sweden, where oxazepam is prescribed by physicians more frequently than diazepam, most prescription forgeries are still for diazepam, presumably reflecting diazepam's greater abuse liability (Bergman and Griffiths 1986; Bliding 1978).

As suggested by their relatively low reinforcing properties, benzodiazepines as a class of drugs are not frequently taken alone for recreational purposes. Although clinicians occasionally see patients who take very high doses of benzodiazepines (without any other drugs or alcohol) for pleasurable purposes, the number of such patients is likely to be relatively small.

The most frequent abuse of benzodiazepines is the ingestion of high doses of these drugs for recreational purposes as part of a pattern of multi-drug abuse (Busto et al. 1986a; DuPont 1988; Edwards et al. 1984; Stitzer et al. 1981). Among drug abusers, benzodiazepines are commonly taken by those who have had a past history of other drug or alcohol abuse (Busto et al. 1983a, 1983b; Ciccone 1987; Jaffe et al. 1983; Perera et al. 1987b).

As part of polydrug abuse, benzodiazepines themselves may be taken to produce euphoria, or they may be used to augment the euphoriant effect of other drugs, especially the opiates. Numerous reports attest to the popularity of benzodiazepines, especially diazepam among opiate abusers (Kleber and Gold 1978; Perera et al. 1987b; Raskin and Bradfor 1975; Woody et al. 1975b); as many as 80% of opiate abusers also take benzodiazepines (Brown and Chaitkin 1981). Benzodiazepines are similarly popular with methadone patients (Budd et al. 1979; Kaul and Davidow 1981; Kleber and Gold 1978; Kokoski et al. 1970; Leifer et al. 1983; Preston et al. 1984; Stitzer et al. 1981; Weddington and Carney 1987; Woody et al. 1975a), in whom the drugs are used to augment the euphoriant effect, as well as to treat anxiety. Cocaine users use benzodiazepines to ease the "crash" of the rapid decline in euphoria. A high percentage of alcohol abusers also take benzodiazepines, ranging from 29%–33% (Busto et al. 1982; Schuckit and Morrissey 1979) to 76% (Ciraulo et al. 1988b; Wiseman and Spencer-Peet 1985). In research studies, high doses of diazepam are clearly reinforcing in subjects with histories of sedative or alcohol abuse (Ciccone 1987; Griffiths et al. 1980; Jaffe et al. 1983). Alcoholics may be at high risk to abuse alprazolam because it has a positive mood effect not seen in nonalcoholics (Ciraulo et al. 1988a). An increasing number of methadone users are also reported now to be augmenting the "high" with alprazolam (Iguchi et al. 1989; Weddington and Carney 1987). Mixed alcohol-benzodiazepine withdrawal produces discontinuance symptoms that are more characteristic of benzodiazepine withdrawal than alcohol withdrawal (Benzer and Cushman 1980; Robinson and Sellers 1982).

Overall, the following conclusions can be drawn regarding abuse of benzodiazepines:

1. Most nonmedically supervised use of benzodiazepines involves the occasional or intermittent use of therapeutic doses for symptomatic relief. This pattern of use is not associated with dose escalation or high-dose recreational abuse.

2. Recreational abuse of benzodiazepines alone is uncommon. Within the drug abuse and alcohol abuse populations, however, benzodiazepines are commonly taken as part of a polysubstance-abuse pattern.
3. As potential drugs of abuse, because of different reinforcing properties one must distinguish among the different benzodiazepines. Present data suggest that diazepam and possibly lorazepam and alprazolam are among the most reinforcing and therefore the most likely to be associated with abuse.

10

Conclusions

GIVEN THE LARGE AMOUNT of benzodiazepines taken throughout the world, concern is justified regarding their appropriate therapeutic use, toxicity, abuse, and risk of inducing a drug-dependent state. The following conclusions are derived from the foregoing review.

1. Although benzodiazepines are widely prescribed and used, most of this use is intermittent, brief, and for purposes of symptom relief. Research survey data indicate that long-term use of benzodiazepines is limited to a relatively small population of patients who take the drugs for legitimate, medically supervised symptom reduction. These patients tend to be older, to have chronic physical as well as psychiatric illness, and to have psychological distress, and these patients report that the drug use is therapeutic. There are no data to suggest that long-term therapeutic use of benzodiazepines by patients commonly leads to dose escalation or to recreational abuse. However, these research survey data concerning patterns of benzodiazepine use do not encompass the period after 1980, when short half-life benzodiazepines were introduced. Clinical perceptions have suggested that use patterns have changed since the introduction of short half-life benzodiazepines. Clinicians have also noted, with increasing frequency, that benzodiazepines may, in fact, not always be used with medical supervision, and that at times doses may be gradually increased. There is a discrepancy between past research survey data and current clinical impressions regarding estimates of benzodiazepine use and dose escalation. This lack of correspondence is between survey data from the past decade when long half-life drugs were most commonly prescribed and current clinical perceptions now that short half-life, more potent benzodiazepines are widely prescribed.

2. A certain small percentage of patients use therapeutic doses of benzodiazepines for self-medication of symptoms. Concern has been expressed in the lay literature and by psychiatrists and

physicians that such use may be inappropriate and potentially hazardous, leading to physiological dependence. Past survey data suggested that the number of people who occasionally self-medicate was small; new survey data are now needed.

3. Physiological dependence on benzodiazepines, as indicated by the appearance of discontinuance symptoms, can develop with therapeutic doses. Duration of treatment determines the onset of dependence when typical therapeutic anxiolytic doses are used; clinically significant dependence indicated by the appearance of discontinuance symptoms usually does not appear before four months of such daily dosing. Dependence may develop sooner when higher antipanic doses are taken daily.

4. Discontinuance symptoms usually develop after abrupt drug termination even of therapeutic doses, but discontinuance symptoms are less frequent and less intense following gradual tapering. The discontinuance symptoms are usually the mirror image of the drug effect; increased anxiety, insomnia, and restlessness are the most common symptoms. There is no difference in the qualitative nature of discontinuance symptoms between long half-life and short half-life benzodiazepines used to treat anxiety.

5. The most immediate discontinuance symptoms tend to be a rebound worsening of the original symptoms. A more severe withdrawal syndrome consists of the appearance of new symptoms, including perceptual hyperacusis, psychosis, cerebellar dysfunction, and seizures. Original symptoms may reappear when the therapeutic medication is withdrawn, and it may be difficult to distinguish recurrence of original symptoms from rebound. Recurrent symptoms tend to persist, whereas rebound lessens after a few days. Concern has been expressed in the recent literature that some withdrawal symptoms may persist for very long periods of time. Research data suggest that most withdrawal symptoms dissipate after approximately 2–4 weeks; an occasional symptom such as tinnitus may persist beyond 4 weeks, but symptoms rarely continue beyond 8 weeks. There are no data to suggest that the effects of benzodiazepines or benzodiazepine withdrawal produce permanent structural or functional brain damage.

6. The onset of discontinuance symptoms is sooner and the symptoms are more intense following abrupt termination of short half-life drugs. In some cases, rebound symptoms appear within hours after the last dose. Rebound symptoms may be so severe that patients prefer to continue benzodiazepine use to avoid the discomfort of discontinuance. Repeated daily administration of

therapeutic doses of benzodiazepines may contribute to the development of dependence, and such long-term use may be a growing public health concern, since the severity of discontinuance symptoms may increase as drugs are taken for longer periods.

7. Clinical experience suggests that the severity of discontinuance symptoms correlates with half-life (being worse with short half-life drugs). The relationship of therapeutic potency to severity of discontinuance that is sometimes observed clinically has not been verified, to date, by research studies.

8. Withdrawal seizures are relatively infrequent but represent the most serious of the withdrawal symptoms. Seizures may be more common after abrupt withdrawal of short half-life, high-potency benzodiazepines, and they are more common in patients who are taking multiple drugs or who have had a history of prior sedative hypnotic use.

9. Various substitute drugs have been used to treat discontinuance symptoms. To date, the most reliable approach to treatment for prevention of discontinuance symptoms is gradual tapering of the benzodiazepine dose. For high-potency, short half-life benzodiazepines (lorazepam, alprazolam, triazolam) this tapering may have to be very gradual.

10. In the CNS, benzodiazepines enhance GABA neurotransmission. The mechanism of benzodiazepine discontinuance symptoms involves the uncovering of the benzodiazepine-GABA receptor. Since GABA is an inhibitory neurotransmitter, the removal of benzodiazepines from these CNS receptor complexes produces an increase (rebound) of arousal symptoms, which may include anxiety, insomnia, and restlessness. It has been hypothesized that the critical variable in the production of discontinuance symptoms is the rate at which the receptor complex is uncovered. The rate of receptor uncovering, in turn, is directly proportional to the rate of decline of benzodiazepine blood level. The rapid reduction of blood and brain levels of short half-life benzodiazepines facilitates this uncovering of receptor sites, resulting in rebound and other symptoms of discontinuance.

11. Sedation and cerebellar dysfunction are the most common benzodiazepine side effects. Benzodiazepines may also impair psychomotor functioning as measured by laboratory tests. Automobile driving is predictably and consistently impaired by *acute* therapeutic doses as well as high doses of benzodiazepines. However, automobile driving is neither predictably nor consistently impaired by *repeated* therapeutic doses of benzodiaze-

pines, and it is likely that therapeutic doses of these drugs, when taken alone, do not play a major role in automobile accidents. Alcohol and advanced age markedly increase the psychomotor toxicity of benzodiazepine, whether taken acutely or on a long-term basis.

12. Benzodiazepines may affect memory function in two ways. With high doses, or with intravenous administration, they may cause an acute anterograde amnesia. When taken orally in therapeutic doses, the impairment typically consists of impaired delayed recall of information that was learned after the drug was taken. In older subjects this memory impairment may be diagnostically confused with aging or progressive dementia. Benzodiazepines may also impair cognitive function in older patients with age-related memory dysfunction or with dementia.

13. Benzodiazepines do not strongly reinforce their own use and are not widely abused drugs. When abuse does occur, it is almost always among persons who are also actively abusing alcohol, opiates, or other sedative hypnotics. In these people, diazepam and alprazolam—the most commonly used benzodiazepines—are the most abused benzodiazepines.

14. This task force suggests the development of guidelines for reasonable prescribing and appropriate clinical management of benzodiazepines, with the advice and concurrence of the treating professions, and vigorous educational interventions aimed at physicians and the general public. The task force also encourages ongoing epidemiological studies of treatment practices and judicious monitoring of prescribing behavior with stepwise feedback to individual prescribers.

11

Prescribing Guidelines

BASED ON THE FOREGOING task force report, several recommendations for prescribing benzodiazepines can be formulated. It should be emphasized, however, that these recommendations are generalizations derived from observations of large numbers of patients and may not apply to a specific clinical situation or to an individual patient. Psychiatrists should always base their prescribing practices on an individual patient's needs rather than on global or general formulations.

When determining whether or not a benzodiazepine should be prescribed, clinicians should now carefully weigh the potential therapeutic benefit against long-term risk of dependency and resulting likelihood of discontinuance symptoms, as well as against acute and chronic drug toxicity. Reduction of acute anxiety panic or insomnia may be remarkably beneficial, and this therapeutic benefit may clearly outweigh any short-term risk of toxicity to benzodiazepines. Clinicians should not be discouraged from prescribing a benzodiazepine when clinically warranted, and they should be reassured that, at least on the short-term basis, for most patients the benefits outweigh the risks. Before prescribing a benzodiazepine, clinicians should carefully evaluate patients for current or past alcohol or other drug dependence.

The question of benefit outweighing risks, however, becomes less clear when therapeutic doses are used over long periods of time, or when greater than therapeutic doses are used for short or even intermediate periods of time. Risks of chronic toxicity, especially cognitive impairment, true physiological dependence, and discontinuance symptoms, are all more likely under the following conditions: 1) high dose, 2) daily dosing of more than 4 months duration, 3) advanced age, 4) current or prior history of sedative hypnotic and/or alcohol dependence including prior chronic benzodiazepine use, and 5) use of high-potency, short half-life benzodiazepines. Alone, or in combination, these risk factors raise serious questions about the wisdom of routine long-term use of benzodiazepines.

There are patients, however, for whom the benefits of ongoing benzodiazepine treatment clearly outweigh the hazards. Typically, these are 1) patients with demonstrable persistent anxiety or dysphoric disorder or anxiety as a component of medical illness that cannot be otherwise treated and 2) patients with chronic panic or agoraphobic disorder when benzodiazepines are deemed the preferred pharmacologic drug by the clinician. Long-term nightly use of benzodiazepines for treatment of insomnia is probably not warranted for most patients and may be especially hazardous in the elderly. However, some elderly patients can sleep only with the assistance of a benzodiazepine. Ongoing use in such patients may be warranted but should be closely supervised. Long-term maintenance adjunctive treatment of psychotic patients who are being treated with neuroleptics, or the use of benzodiazepines to treat depressive symptoms, has not yet been sufficiently demonstrated to be efficacious to become standard ongoing therapy.

In summary, therefore, clinicians should endeavor to use the lowest benzodiazepine doses that are therapeutic and treat for the briefest period of time as indicated by the patient's own clinical condition. Ongoing daily maintenance treatment of benzodiazepines should be decided on a case-by-case basis, and clinicians should regularly reevaluate these patients in order to ensure that continued benzodiazepine use is therapeutic and warranted. Unsupervised long-term benzodiazepine use is not recommended. Special caution should be taken when benzodiazepines are prescribed to the elderly or to those with a current or prior history of substance abuse or dependence.

References

Abernethy DR, Greenblatt DJ, Shader RI: Treatment of diazepam withdrawal syndrome with propranolol. Ann Intern Med 94: 354–355, 1981

Abernethy DR, Greenblatt DJ, Shader RI: Benzodiazepines in clinical practice, in Recent Advances in Clinical Therapeutics. Edited by Vetiv JZ, Bianchine JR. New York, Grune and Stratton, 1983, pp 143–157

Acuda SW, Muhangi J: Diazepam addiction in Kenya. East Afr Med J 56:76–79, 1979

Adam K, Oswald I, Shapiro C: Effects of loprazolam and of triazolam on sleep and overnight urinary cortisol. Psychopharmacology 82:389–394, 1984

Adam K, Adamson L, Brezinova V, et al: Nitrazepam: lastingly effective but trouble on withdrawal. Br Med J 1:1558–1560, 1976

Agrawal P: Diazepam addiction: a case report. Canadian Psychiatric Association Journal 23:35–37, 1978

Albeck JH: Withdrawal and detoxification from benzodiazepine dependence: a potential role for clonazepam. J Clin Psychiatry 48:10S, 1987

Allgulander C: Dependence on sedative and hypnotic drugs: a comparative clinical and social study. Acta Psychiatr Scand [Suppl] 270S:7–101, 1978

Allgulander C, Borg S: A case report: a delerious abstinence syndrome associated with clorazepate (Tranxiline). Br J Addict 73:175–177, 1978

Angus WR, Romney DM: The effect of diazepam on patients' memory. J Clin Psychopharmacol 4:203–206, 1984

Anonymous: Some problems with benzodiazepines. Drug and Therapeutics Bulletin 23:21–23, 1985

Aranko K, Mattila MJ, Seppala T: Development of tolerance and cross-tolerance to the psychomotor actions of lorazepam and diazepam in man. Br J Clin Pharmacol 15:545–552, 1983

Aranko K, Mattila MJ, Bordignon D: Psychomotor effects of alprazolam and diazepam during acute and subacute treatment, and during the follow-up phase. Acta Pharmacologica et Toxicologica 56:364–372, 1985

Ashton H: Benzodiazepine withdrawal: an unfinished story. Br Med J 88:1135–1140, 1984

Athinarayanan P, Pierog SH, Nigam SK, et al: Chlordiazepoxide withdrawal in the neonate. Am J Obstet Gynecol 124:212–213, 1976

Ayd F: Benzodiazepines: dependence and withdrawal. JAMA 242: 1401, 1979

Ayd F: Diazepam dependency and withdrawal. Current Psychiatric Therapy 20:263–274, 1981

Balmer R, Battegay R, von Marschall R: Long-term treatment with diazepam: investigation of consumption habits and the interaction between psychotherapy and psychopharmacotherapy: a prospective study. Pharmacopsychiatry 16:221–234, 1981

Balter MB: Clinical epidemiology of treatment with prescription medications with dependent liability. Faculty Presentation at Martebello Conference on Development of Educational Strategies for Prescribing Drugs with Depdendence Liability: Optimal Therapy the Goal, Montebello, Quebec, Canada, June 2–3, 1988

Balter MB, Manheimer DI, Mellinger GE, et al: A cross-national comparison of anti-anxiety/sedative drug use. Curr Med Res Opin 8S:5–20, 1984

Bargmann E, Wolfe SM, Levin J, et al: Stopping Valium. Washington, DC, Public Citizen's Health Research Group, 1982

Barten HH: Toxic psychosis with transient dysmnestic syndrome following withdrawal from Valium. Am J Psychiatry 121:1210–1211, 1965

Barton DF: More on lorazepam withdrawal. Drug Intell Clin Pharm 15:487–488, 1981

Bastos ML, Galante L: Toxicological findings in victims of traumatic deaths. J Forensic Sci 21:176–186, 1976

Beers M, Avorn J, Soremerai SB: Psychoactive medication use in intermediate-care residents. JAMA 260:3016–3020, 1988

Benzer D, Cushman P: Alcohol and benzodiazepines: withdrawal syndromes. Alcoholism: Clinical and Experimental Research 4:243–247, 1980

Berg SW, Fryback JT, Goldenbaum DM, et al: The Study of Possible Influence of Licit and Illicit Drugs on Driver Behavior. Department of Transportation Report DOT HS-800 613. Washington, DC, US Department of Transportation, 1971

Bergman U, Griffiths RR: Relative abuse of diazepam and oxazepam: prescription forgeries and theft/loss reports in Sweden. Drug and Alcohol Dependence 16:293–301, 1986

Berlin RM, Conell LJ: Withdrawal symptoms after long-term treatment with therapeutic doses of flurazepam: a case report. Am J Psychiatry 140:488–490, 1983

Betts TA, Birtle J: Effect of two hypnotic drugs on actual driving performance next morning. Br Med J 285:852, 1982

Betts TA, Clayton AB, Mackay GM: Effects of four commonly used tranquillizers on low-speed driving performance tests. Br Med J 4:580–584, 1972

Bixler EO, Scharf MB, Soldatos CR, et al: Effects of hypnotics on memory. Life Sci 25:1379–1388, 1979

Bixler EO, Kales JD, Kales A, et al: Rebound insomnia and elimination half-life: assessment of individual subject response. J Clin Pharmacol 25:115–124, 1985

Blackburn RR, Woodhouse EJ: A Comparison of Drug Use in Driver Fatalities and Similarly Exposed Drivers. US Department of Transportation Report DOT HS-802 488. Washington, DC, US Department of Transportation, 1977

Bliding A: The abuse potential of benzodiazepines with special reference to oxazepam. Acta Psychiatr Scand 274S:111S–116S, 1978

Bliwise DL, Seidel WF, Cohen SA, et al: Profile of mood changes during and after 5 weeks of nightly triazolam administration. J Clin Psychiatry 49:349–355, 1988

Block RI, Berchou R: Alprazolam and lorazepam effects on memory acquisition and retrieval processes. Pharmacol Biochem Behav 20:233–241, 1984

Bo O, Haffner JFW, Landard O, et al: Ethanol and diazepam as causative agents in road traffic accidents, in Alcohol, Drugs, and Traffic Safety: Proceedings of the Sixth International Conference (September 1974). Edited by Israelstam S, Lambert S. Toronto, Addiction Research Foundation, 1975, pp 439–448

Bond AJ, James DC, Lader MH: Sedative effects on physiological and psychological measures in anxious patients. Psychol Med 4:374–380, 1974

Böning J: Benzodiazepine dependence: clinical and neurobiological aspects, in Chronic Treatments in Neuropsychiatry. Edited by Kemali D, Racagni G. New York, Raven Press, 1985, pp 185–192

Bonnet MH, Kramer M: The interaction of age, performance, and hypnotics in the sleep of insomniacs. J Am Geriatr Soc 29:508–512, 1981

Bornstein RA, Watson GD, Pawluk LK: Effects of chronic benzodiazepine administration and neuropsychological performance. Clin Neuropharmacol 8:357–361, 1985

Borrow S, Idzikowski C: Flurazepam improves sleep but impairs psychomotor performance. Waking Sleeping 3:69–70, 1979

Bowden CL, Fisher JG: Safety and efficacy of long-term diazepam therapy. South Med J 73:1581–1584, 1980

Breier A, Charney DS, Nelson JC: Seizures induced by abrupt discontinuation of alprazolam. Am J Psychiatry 141:1606–1607, 1984

Brewin R: Businessmen hooked on valium. Dun's Review, January 1978, pp 44–46

Brown BS, Chaitkin L: Use of stimulant/depressant drugs by drug abuse clients in selected metropolitan areas. Int J Addict 16:1473–1490, 1981

Brown J, Lewis V, Brown MW, et al: Amnesic effects of intravenous diazepam and lorazepam. Experientia (Basel) 34:501–502, 1978

Brown J, Brown MW, Bowes JB: A comparison between benzodiazepine (lorazepam)-induced amnesia and that of the hippicampal syndrome. Neurosci Lett 10S:92S, 1982

Brown SS, Dundee JW: Clinical studies of induction agents, XXV: diazepam. Br J Anaesth 40:108–112, 1968

Browne JL, Hauge KJ: A review of alprazolam withdrawal. Drug Intell Clin Pharm 20:837–841, 1986

Budd RD, Walkin E, Jain NV, et al: Frequency of use of diazepam in individuals on probation and in methadone maintenance programs. Am J Drug Alcohol Abuse 6:511–514, 1979

Burrows G: Short-acting vs. long-acting benzodiazepine discontinuation effects in panic disorders. J Psychiatr Res (in press)

Busto U, Sellers EM: Pharmacokinetic determinants of drug abuse and dependence: a conceptual perspective. Clinical Pharmacokinetics 11:144–153, 1986

Busto U, Sellers EM, Sisson B, et al: Benzodiazepine use and abuse in alcoholics. Clin Pharmacol Ther 31:207–208, 1982

Busto U, Naranjo CA, Cappell H, et al: Patterns of benzodiazepine abuse. Clin Pharmacol Ther 33:237, 1983a

Busto U, Simpkins J, Sellers EM, et al: Objective determination of benzodiazepine use and abuse in alcoholics. Br J Addict 78: 429–435, 1983b

Busto U, Sellers EM, Naranjo CA, et al: Patterns of benzodiazepine abuse and dependence. Br J Addict 81:87–94, 1986a

Busto U, Sellers EM, Naranjo CA, et al: Withdrawal reaction after long-term therapeutic use of benzodiazepines. N Engl J Med

315:854–859, 1986b

Busto U, Fornazzari L, Naranjo CA: Protracted tinnitus after discontinuation of long-term therapeutic use of benzodiazepines. J Clin Psychopharmacol 8:359–362, 1988

Cant G: Valiumania. The New York Times Magazine, February 1976, pp 34–44

Carney MWP, Ellis PF: A policy on benzodiazepines (response to letter). Lancet 2:1406, 1987

Carskadon MA, Seidel WF, Greenblatt DJ, et al: Daytime carryover of triazolam and flurazepam in elderly insomniacs. Sleep 5: 361–371, 1982

Catalan J, Gath DH, Bond A, et al: General practice patients on long-term psychotropic drugs: a controlled investigation. Br J Psychiatry 152:399–405, 1988

Charney DS, Heninger GR, Sternberg DE, et al: Abrupt discontinuation of tricyclic antidepressant drugs: evidence for noradrenergic hyperactivity. Br J Psychiatry 141:377–386, 1982

Christensen JD: Tolerance development with chlordiazepoxide in relation to the plasma levels of the parent compound and its main metabolites in mice. Acta Pharmacologica et Toxicologica 33:262–272, 1973

Church MW, Johnson LC: Mood and performance of poor sleepers during repeated use of flurazepam. Psychopharmacology 61: 309–316, 1979

Ciccone PE: Misuse and abuse of benzodiazepines (letter). Am J Psychiatry 144:1246–1247, 1987

Cimbura G, Lucas DM, Bennett RC, et al: Incidence and toxicological aspects of drugs detected in 484 fatally injured drivers and pedestrians in Ontario. J Forensic Sci 27:855–867, 1982

Ciraulo DA, Barnhill JG, Greenblatt DJ, et al: Abuse liability and clinical pharmacokinetics of alprazolam in alcoholic men. J Clin Psychiatry 49:333–337, 1988a

Ciraulo D, Sands BF, Shader RI: Critical review of liability for benzodiazepine abuse among alcoholics. Am J Psychiatry 145: 1501–1506, 1988b

Clare AW: Diazepam, alcohol, and barbiturate abuse. Br Med J 4:340, 1971

Clark EO, Glanzer M, Turndorf H: The pattern of memory loss resulting from intravenously administered diazepam. Arch Neurol 36:296–300, 1979

Clarke PRF, Eccersley PS, Frisby JP, et al: The amnesic effect of diazepam (Valium). Br J Anaesth 42:690–697, 1970

Cohen LS, Heller VL, Rosenbaum JF: Treatment guidelines for psychotropic drug use in pregnancy. Psychosomatics 30:25–

33, 1989

Cohen SI: Are benzodiazepines useful in anxiety? (letter). Lancet 2:1080, 1987

Cohn JB, Noble EP: Effect of withdrawing treatment after long-term administration of alprazolam, lorazepam, or placebo in patients with an anxiety disorder. Psychopharmacol Bull 19:751–752, 1983

Cohn JB, Wilcox CS: Long-term comparison of alprazolam, lorazepam and placebo in patients with an anxiety disorder. Pharmacotherapy 4:93–98, 1984

Cook PJ, Huggett A, Graham PR, et al: Hypnotic accumulation and hangover in elderly inpatients: a controlled double-blind study of temazepam and nitrazepam. Br Med J 286:100–102, 1983

Covi L, Park LC, Lipman RS, et al: Factors affecting withdrawal response to certain minor tranquilizers, in Drug Abuse: Social and Psychopharmacological Aspects. Edited by Cole JO, Wittenborn JR. Springfield, IL, Charles C Thomas, 1969, pp 93–108

Covi L, Lipman RS, Pattison JH, et al: Length of treatment with anxiolytic sedatives and response to their sudden withdrawal. Acta Psychiatr Scand 49:51–64, 1973

Cowen PJ, Nutt DJ: Abstinence symptoms after withdrawal of tranquillizing drugs: is there a common neurochemical mechanism? Lancet 2:360–362, 1982

Crawley JN, Marangos PJ, Stivers J, et al: Chronic clonazepam administration induces benzodiazepine receptor subsensitivity. Neuropharmacology 21:85–89, 1982

Crooks J: Aging and drug disposition: pharmacodynamics. J Chronic Dis 36:85–90, 1983

Curran HV, Schiwy W, Lader M: Differential amnesic properties of benzodiazepines: a dose-response comparison of two drugs with similar elimination half-lives. Psychopharmacology 92:358–364, 1987

De Bard ML: Diazepam withdrawal syndrome: a case with psychosis, seizure, and coma. Am J Psychiatry 136:104–105, 1979

De Gier JJ, Hart BJT, Nelemans FA, et al: Psychomotor performance and real driving performance of outpatients receiving diazepam. Psychopharmacology 73:340–344, 1981

de la Fuente JR, Rosenbaum AH, Martin HR, et al: Lorazepam-related withdrawal seizures. Mayo Clin Proc 55:190–192, 1980

Dement WC: Daytime sleepiness/alertness levels: measurements and sleep-related determinants. Paper presented at the Annual Meeting of the American College of Neuropsychopharmacology, Washington, DC, December 9, 1986

De Wit H, Johanson CE, Uhlenhuth EH: Reinforcing properties of lorazepam in normal volunteer subjects. Drug and Alcohol Dependence 13:21–31, 1984a

De Wit H, Johanson CE, Uhlenhuth EH: The dependence potential of benzodiazepines. Curr Med Res Opin 8S:48S–52S, 1984b

De Wit H, Uhlenhuth EH, Johanson CE: Lack of preference for flurazepam in normal volunteers. Pharmacology Biochemistry and Behavior 21:865–869, 1985

De Wit H, Uhlenhuth EH, Hedeker D, et al: Lack of preference for diazepam in anxious volunteers. Arch Gen Psychiatry 43:533–541, 1986

Desjardins PJ, Beaver WT: Psychomotor and memory impairment after intravenous diazepam, meperidine plus diazepam, or placebo in oral surgery patients. Clin Pharmacol Ther 31:216–217, 1982

Desjardins PJ, Moerschbaecher JM, Thompson DM: Intravenous diazepam in humans: effects on acquisition and performance of response chains. Pharmacol Biochem Behav 17:1055–1059, 1982

Dietch J: The nature and extent of benzodiazepine abuse: an overview of recent literature. Hosp Community Psychiatry 34:1139–1145, 1983

Dietch JT, Jennings RK: Aggressive dyscontrol in patients treated with benzodiazepines. J Clin Psychiatry 49:184–188, 1988

Dimascio A, Barrett J: Comparative effects of oxazepam in "high" and "low" anxious student volunteers. Psychosomatics 6:298–302, 1965

Dimascio A, Gardos G, Harmatz J, et al: Tybamate: an examination of its actions in "high" and "low" anxious normals. Diseases of the Nervous System 30:758–763, 1969

Doongaji DB, Sheth A, Apte JS, et al: Clobazam versus diazepam—a double-blind study in anxiety neurosis. J Clin Pharmacol 18:358–364, 1978

Dundee JW, Haslett WHK: The benzodiazepines: a review of their actions and uses relative to anaesthetic practice. Br J Anaesth 42:217–234, 1970

Dundee JW, Pandit SK: Anterograde amnesic effects of pethidine, hyoscine, and diazepam in adults. Br J Pharmacol 44:140–144, 1972

DuPont RL: Substance abuse. JAMA 256:2114–2116, 1986

DuPont RL: Abuse of benzodiazepines: the problems and the solutions. Am J Drug Alcohol Abuse 14S:1–69, 1988

Dysken MW, Chan CH: Diazepam withdrawal psychosis: a case report. Am J Psychiatry 134:573, 1977

Edwards JG, Cantopher T, Olivieri S: Dependence on psychotropic drugs: an overview. Postgrad Med J 60S:29S, 1984

Ehrlich C: Halcion nightmare: the frightening truth about America's favorite sleeping pill. California, September 1988a, pp 60–119

Ehrlich C: Halcion: prescription for trouble? California, October 1988b, pp 74–77

Einarson TR: Lorazepam withdrawal seizures. Lancet 1:151, 1980

Einarson TR: Oxazepam withdrawal convulsions. Drug Intell Clin Pharm 15:487–488, 1981

Ellinwood EH, Nikaido AM: Perceptual-neurometer pharmacodynamics of psychotropic drugs, in Psychopharmacology: The Third Generation in Progress. Edited by Meltzer HY. New York, Raven Press, 1987, pp 1457–1466

Erwin CW, Linnoila M, Hartwell J, et al: Effects of buspirone and diazepam, alone and in combination with alcohol on skilled performance and evoked potential. J Clin Psychopharmacol 6:199–207, 1986

Fabre LF, McLendon DM, Stephens AG: Comparison of the therapeutic effect, tolerance, and safety of ketazolam and diazepam administered for six months to outpatients with chronic anxiety neurosis. J Int Med Res 9:191–198, 1981

Ferholt JB, Stone WN: Severe delirium after abrupt withdrawal of thiothixene in a chronic schizophrenic inpatient. J Nerv Ment Dis 150:400–403, 1970

File SE: Rapid development of tolerance to the sedative effects of lorazepam and triazolam in rats. Psychopharmacology 73:240–245, 1981

File SE: Development and retention of tolerance to the sedative effects of chlordiazepoxide: role of apparatus cues. Eur J Pharmacol 81:637–643, 1982a

File SE: Recovery from lorazepam tolerance and the effects of a benzodiazepine antagonist (RO 15-1788) on the development of tolerance. Psychopharmacology 77:284–288, 1982b

Finkle BS, Biasotti AA, Crim M, et al: The occurrence of some drugs and toxic agents encountered in drinking driver investigations. J Forensic Sci 13:236–245, 1968

Fisher RS: Multidisciplinary Accident Investigation. Department of Transportation Report DOT HS-800 782. Washington, DC, US Department of Transportation, 1973

Fleischhacker WW, Barnas C, Hackenberg B: Epidemiology of benzodiazepine dependence. Acta Psychiatr Scand 74:80–83, 1986

Floyd JB Jr, Murphy CM: Hallucinations following withdrawal of valium. J Ky Med Assoc 74:549–550, 1976

Fontaine R, Chouinard G, Annable A: Rebound anxiety in anxious patients after abrupt withdrawal of benzodiazepine treatment. Am J Psychiatry 141:848–852, 1984

Fontaine R, Chouinard G, Annable L: Efficacy and withdrawal of two potent benzodiazepines: bromazepam and lorazepam. Psychopharmacology Bull 21:91–92, 1985

Foy A, Drinkwater V, March S, et al: Confusion after admission to hospital in elderly patients using benzodiazepines. Br Med J 293:1072, 1986

Frith CD, Richardson JTE, Samuel M, et al: The effects of intravenous diazepam and hyoscine upon human memory. Q J Exp Psychol [A] 36A:133–144, 1984

Fruensgaard K: Withdrawal psychosis: a study of 30 consecutive cases. Acta Psychiatr Scand 53:105–118, 1976

Fyer AJ, Liebowitz MR, Gorman JM, et al: Discontinuation of alprazolam treatment in panic patients. Am J Psychiatry 144:303–308, 1987

Fyer AJ, Liebowitz JM, Gorman JM, et al: Effects of clonidine on alprazolam discontinuation in panic patients: a pilot study. J Clin Psychopharmacol 8:270–274, 1988

Gallager DW, Lakoski JM, Gonsalves SF, et al: Chronic benzodiazepine treatment decreases post-synaptic GABA sensitivity. Nature 208:74–77, 1984

Gardner DL, Cowdry RW: Alprazolam-induced dyscontrol in borderline personality disorder. Am J Psychiatry 142:98–100, 1985

Garriott JC, Latman N: Drug detection in cases of "driving under the influence." J Forensic Sci 21:398–415, 1976

Garriott JC, Dimaio VJM, Zumwalt RE, et al: Incidence of drugs and alcohol in fatally injured motor vehicle drivers. J Forensic Sci 22:383–389, 1977

Garriott JC, Dimaio VJM, Rodriguez RG: Detection of cannabinoids in homicide victims and motor vehicle fatalities. J Forensic Sci 31:1274–1282, 1986

Garvey MJ, Tollefson GD: Prevalence of misuse of prescribed benzodiazepines in patients with primary anxiety disorder or major depression. Am J Psychiatry 143:1601–1603, 1986

Ghoneim MM, Mewaldt SP: Studies on human memory: the interactions of diazepam, scopolamine, and physostigmine. Psychopharmacology 52:1–6, 1977

Ghoneim MM, Mewaldt SP, Thatcher JW: The effect of diazepam and fentanyl on mental, psychomotor, and electroencephalographic functions and their rate of recovery. Psychopharmacologia 44:61–66, 1975

Ghoneim MM, Mewaldt SP, Berie JL, et al: Memory and performance effects of single and 3-week administration of diazepam. Psychopharmacology 73:147–151, 1981

Ghoneim MM, Hinrichs JV, Mewaldt SP: Dose response analysis of the behavioral effects of diazepam, I: Learning and memory. Psychopharmacology 82:291–295, 1984

Giles HG, MacLeod SM, Wright JR, et al: Influence of age and previous use of diazepam dosage required for endoscopy. Can Med Assoc J 118:513–514, 1978

Gill TS, Guram MS, Geber WF: Comparative study of the teratogenic effects of chlordiazepoxide and diazepam in the fetal hamster. Life Sci 29:2141–2147, 1981

Gillin JC, Spinweber CL, Johnson LC: Rebound insomnia: a critical review. J Clin Psychopharmacol 9:161–172, 1989

Golombok S, Higgitt A, Fonagy P, et al: A follow-up study of patients treated for benzodiazepine dependence. Br J Med Psychol 60:141–149, 1987

Golombok S, Moodley P, Lader M: Cognitive impairment in long-term benzodiazepine users. Psychol Med 18:365–374, 1988

Gordon B: I'm Dancing as Fast as I Can. New York, Harper & Row, 1979

Gordon EB: Addiction to diazepam (Valium). Br Med J 1:112, 1967

Granek E, Baker SP, Abbey H, et al: Medications and diagnoses in relation to falls in long-term care facilities. J Am Geriatr Soc 35:503–511, 1987

Greenblatt DJ, Shader RI: Benzodiazepines in clinical practice. New York, Raven Press, 1974a

Greenblatt DJ, Shader RI: Benzodiazepines: part I. N Engl J Med 291:1011–1015, 1974b

Greenblatt DJ, Shader RI: Dependence, tolerance, and addiction to benzodiazepines: clinical and pharmacokinetic considerations. Drug Metab Rev 8:13–28, 1978

Greenblatt DJ, Shader RI, Abernethy DR: Current status of benzodiazepines: part I. N Engl J Med 309:354–358, 1983a

Greenblatt DJ, Shader RI, Abernethy DR: Current status of benzodiazepines: part II. N Engl J Med 309:410–416, 1983b

Greenblatt DJ, Harmatz JS, Zinny MA, et al: Effect of gradual withdrawal on the rebound sleep disorder after discontinuation of triazolam. N Engl J Med 317:722–728, 1987a

Greenblatt DJ, Miller LG, Shader RI: Clonazepam pharmacokinetics, brain uptake, and receptor interaction. J Clin Psychiatry 48S:10S, 1987b

Griffiths RR, Ator NA: Benzodiazepine self-administration in animals and humans: a comprehensive literature review. Natl Inst Drug Abuse Res Monogr Ser 33:22–36, 1981

Griffiths RR, Roache JD: Abuse liability of benzodiazepines: a review of human studies evaluating subjective and/or reinforcing effects, in Benzodiazepines: Standards of Use in Clinical Practice. Edited by Smith DE, Wesson DR. Boston, MTP Press, 1985, pp 209–226

Griffiths RR, Sannerud CA: Abuse of and dependence on benzodiazepines and other anxiolytic/sedative drugs, in Psychopharmacology, The Third Generation of Progress. Edited by Meltzer H. New York, Raven Press, 1987, pp 1535–1541

Griffiths RR, Wolf B: Relative abuse liability of different benzodiazepines in drug abusers (unpublished manuscript), 1989

Griffiths RR, Bigelow G, Liebson I: Human drug self-administration: double-blind comparison of pentobarbital, diazepam, chlorpromazine and placebo. J Pharmacol Exp Ther 210:301–310, 1979

Griffiths RR, Bigelow GE, Liebson I, et al: Drug preference in humans: double-blind choice comparison of pentobarbital, diazepam, and placebo. J Pharmacol Exp Ther 215:649–661, 1980

Griffiths RR, Lukas SE, Bradford D, et al: Self-injection of barbiturates and benzodiazepines in baboons. Psychopharmacology 75:101–109, 1981

Griffiths RR, McLeod DR, Bigelow GE, et al: Relative abuse liability of diazepam and oxazepam: behavioral and subjective dose effects. Psychopharmacology 84:147–154, 1984

Griffiths RR, Lamb RJ, Ator NA, et al: Relative abuse liability of triazolam: experimental assessment in animals and humans. Neurosci Biobehav Rev 9:133–151, 1985

Grove-White IG, Kelman GR: Effect of methohexitone, diazepam, and sodium 4-hydroxybutyrate on short-term memory. Br J Anaesth 43:113–116, 1971

Haefely W: Biological basis of drug-induced tolerance, rebound, and dependence: contribution of recent research on benzodiazepines. Pharmacopsychiatry 19:353–361, 1986

Haigh JRM, Feely M: Tolerance to the anticonvulsant effect of benzodiazepines. Trends in Pharmacologic Sciences 9:361–366, 1988

Hakkinen S: Traffic accidents and psychomotor test performance: a follow-up study. Mod Probl Pharmacopsychiatry 1:51–56, 1976

Hanna SM: A case of oxazepam (Serenid D) dependence. Br J Psychiatry 120:443–445, 1972

Harrison M, Busto U, Naranjo CA, et al: Diazepam tapering in detoxification for high-dose benzodiazepine abuse. Clin Pharmacol Ther 36:527–533, 1984

Hartley LR, Spencer J, Williamson J: Anxiety, diazepam, and retrieval from semantic memory. Psychopharmacology 76:291–293, 1982

Haskell D: Withdrawal of diazepam (letter). JAMA 233:135, 1975

Haskell D: Withdrawal of diazepam (letter). JAMA 235:597, 1976

Healey M, Pickens R, Meisch R, et al: Effects of clorazepate, diazepam, lorazepam, and placebo on human memory. J Clin Psychiatry 44:436–439, 1983

Heisterkamp DV, Cohen PJ: The effect of intravenous premedication with lorazepam (Ativan), pentobarbitone, or diazepam on recall. Br J Anaesth 47:70–81, 1975

Heritch AJ, Capwell R, Roy-Byrne PP: A case of psychosis and delirium following withdrawal from triazolam. J Clin Psychiatry 48:168–169, 1987

Herman JB: Comparing alprazolam and clonazepam in the treatment of panic disorders. Currents 7:5–10, 1988

Herman JB, Brotman AW, Rosenbaum JF: Rebound anxiety in panic disorder patients treated with shorter-acting benzodiazepines. J Clin Psychiatry 48S:22–26, 1987

Higgitt AC, Lader MH, Fonagy P: Clinical management of benzodiazepine dependence. Br Med J 291:688–690, 1985

Himmelhoch JM: Benzodiazepine dependence: a spectrum of clinical syndromes, in Anxiety Disorders: An International Update (proceedings). New York, Academy Professional Information Services, 1986, pp 53–64

Hindmarch I: A preliminary study of the effects of repeated doses of clobazam on aspects of performance, arousal, and behavior in a group of anxiety rated volunteers. Eur J Clin Pharmacol 16:17–21, 1979a

Hindmarch I: Some aspects of the effects of clobazam on human psychomotor performance. Br J Clin Pharmacol 7S:77S–82S, 1979b

Hindmarch I, Gudgeon AC: The effects of clobazam and lorazepam on aspects of psychomotor performance and car handling ability. Br J Clin Pharmacol 10:145–150, 1980

Hindmarch I, Subhan Z: The effect of midazolam in conjunction with alcohol on sleep, pscyhomotor performance, and car driving ability. Int J Clin Pharmacol Res 3:323–329, 1983

Hindmarch I, Hanks GW, Hewett AJ: Clobazam, a 1,5-benzodiazepine, and car-driving ability. Br J Clin Pharmacol 4:573–578, 1977

Hinrichs JV, Mewaldt SP, Ghoneim MM, et al: Diazepam and learning: assessment of acquisition deficits. Pharmacol Biochem

Behav 17:165–170, 1982

Hinrichs JV, Ghoneim MM, Mewaldt SP: Diazepam and memory: retrograde facilitation produced by interference reduction. Psychopharmacology 84:158–162, 1984

Hollister LE: Withdrawal from benzodiazepine therapy. JAMA 237: 1432, 1977

Hollister LE: Recent media coverage inflates fear of using benzodiazepines. Clinical Psychiatry News 8:1–38, 1980

Hollister LE: Pharmacology and pharmacokinetics of the minor tranquilizers. Psychiatric Annals 2:26–31, 1981

Hollister LE, Motzenbacker F, Degan R: Withdrawal reactions from chlordiazepoxide ("Librium"). Psychopharmacology 2:63–68, 1961

Hollister LE, Conley FK, Britt RH, et al: Long-term use of diazepam. JAMA 246:1568–1570, 1981

Holmgren P, Loch E, Schuberth J: Drugs in motorists traveling Swedish roads: on-the-road detection of intoxicated drivers and screening for drugs in these offenders. Forensic Sci Int 27:57–65, 1985

Honkanen R, Ertama L, Linnoila M, et al: Role of drugs in traffic accidents. Br Med J 281:1309–1312, 1980

Howe JG: Lorazepam withdrawal seizures. Br Med J 280:1163–1164, 1980

Iguchi MY, Griffiths RR, Bickel WK, et al: Relative abuse liability of benzodiazepines in methadone-maintained populations in three cities, in Problems of Drug Dependence. Edited by Harris LS. Washington, DC, Department of Health and Human Services, 1989

Jaffe JH, Ciraulo DA, Nies A, et al: Abuse potential of halazepam and of diazepam in patients recently treated for acute alcohol withdrawal. Clin Pharmacol Ther 34:623–630, 1983

Jerkovich G, Preskorn S: Failure of buspirone to protect against lorazepam withdrawal symptoms. JAMA 258:204–205, 1987

Jick H, Hunter JR, Dinan BJ, et al: Sedating drugs and automobile accidents leading to hospitalization. Am J Public Health 71: 1399–1400, 1981

Johanson CE, Schuster CR: The effects of RO 15-1788 on anxiolytic self-administration in the rhesus monkey. Pharmacol Biochem Behav 24:855–859, 1986

Johanson CE, Uhlenhuth EH: Drug preference and mood in humans: diazepam. Psychopharmacology 71:269–273, 1980

Johnson LC, Chernik DA: Sedative-hypnotics and human performance. Psychopharmacology 76:101–113, 1982

Jones DM, Jones MEL, Lewis MJ, et al: Drugs and human memory:

effects of low doses of nitrazepam and hyoscine on retention. Br J Clin Pharmacol 7:479–483, 1979

Juergens SM, Morse RM: Alprazolam dependence in seven patients. Am J Psychiatry 145:625–627, 1988

Kahan BB, Haskett RF: Lorazepam withdrawal and seizures. Am J Psychiatry 141:1011–1012, 1984

Kales A, Kales JD: Sleep laboratory studies of hypnotic drugs: efficacy and withdrawal effects. J Clin Psychopharmacol 3:140–150, 1983

Kales A, Bixler EO, Tan TL, et al: Chronic hypnotic use: ineffectiveness, drug-withdrawal insomnia and dependence. JAMA 227: 513–517, 1974

Kales A, Scharf MB, Kales JD: Rebound insomnia: a new clinical syndrome. Science 201:1039–1041, 1978

Kales A, Scharf MB, Kales JD, et al: Rebound insomnia: a potential hazard following withdrawal of certain benzodiazepines. JAMA 241:1692–1695, 1979

Kales A, Bixler EO, Soldatos CR, et al: Quazepam and flurazepam: long-term use and extended withdrawal. Clin Pharmacol Ther 30:782–788, 1982

Kales A, Soldatos CR, Bixler EO, et al: Early morning insomnia with rapidly eliminated benzodiazepines. Science 220:95–97, 1983a

Kales A, Soldatos CR, Bixler EO, et al: Rebound insomnia and rebound anxiety: a review. Pharmacology 26:121–137, 1983b

Kantor SJ: A difficult alprazolam withdrawal. J Clin Psychopharmacol 6:124–125, 1986

Kaul B, Davidow B: Drug abuse patterns of patients on methadone treatment in New York City. Am J Drug Alcohol Abuse 8:17–25, 1981

Keshavian MS, Crammer JL: Clonidine in benzodiazepine withdrawal. Lancet 1:1325–1326, 1985

Khan A, Joyce P, Jones AV: Benzodiazepine withdrawal syndromes. N Z Med J 92:94–96, 1980

Kielholz P, Goldberg L, Obersteg JM, et al: Driving tests to determine the impairment of driving ability by alcohol, tranquilizers, and hypnotics. Forensic Psychiatry 1:150–164, 1972

King MB, Rodrigo EK, Williams P: Health of long-term benzodiazepine users. Br Med J 296:603–606, 1988

Kleber HD, Gold MS: Use of psychotropic drugs in treatment of methadone maintained narcotic addicts. Ann NY Acad Sci 311:81–98, 1978

Klein E, Uhde TW, Post RM: Preliminary evidence for the utility of carbamazepine in alprazolam withdrawal. Am J Psychiatry 143:235–236, 1986, 1986

Kleinknecht RA, Donaldson D: A review of the effects of diazepam on cognitive and psychomotor performance. J Nerv Ment Dis 161:399–411, 1975

Kochansky GE, Salzman C, Shader RI, et al: The differential effects of oxazepam and chlordiazepoxide upon hostility in small group setting. Am J Psychiatry 36:861–863, 1975

Kokoski RJ, Hamner S, Shiplet M: Detection of the use of methaqualone and benzodiazepines in urine screening program. Int J Addict 5:1073–1078, 1970

Kramer M, Schoen LS: Problems in the use of long-acting hypnotics in older patients. J Clin Psychiatry 45:176–177, 1984

Krantz P, Wannerberg O: Occurrence of barbiturate, benzodiazepine, meprobamate, methaqualone, and phenothiazine in car occupants killed in traffic accidents in the south of Sweden. Forensic Sci Int 18:141–147, 1981

Lader M: Benzodiazepine withdrawal states, in Benzodiazepine Divided. Edited by Trimble MR. New York, John Wiley and Sons, 1983a, pp 17–32

Lader M: Dependence on benzodiazepines. J Clin Psychiatry 44:121–127, 1983b

Lader M: Benzodiazepine dependence. Prog Neuropsychopharmacol Biol Psychiatry 8:85–95, 1984

Lader M: Clinical pharmacology of benzodiazepines. Annu Rev Med 38:19–28, 1987a

Lader M: Long-term anxiolytic therapy: the issue of drug withdrawal. J Clin Psychiatry 48:12–16, 1987b

Lader M, File S: The biological basis of benzodiazepine dependence (editorial). Psychol Med 17:539–547, 1987

Lader M, Petursson H: Abuse liability of anxiolytics, in Anxiolytics: Neurochemical, Behavioral, and Clinical Perspectives. Edited by Malick JB, Enna SJ, Yamamura HI. New York, Raven Press, 1983a, pp 201–214

Lader M, Petursson H: Long-term effects of benzodiazepines. Neuropharmacology 22:527–533, 1983b

Lader M, Petursson H: Rational use of anxiolytic/sedative drugs. Drugs 25:514–528, 1983c

Lader M, Curry S, Baker WJ: Physiological and psychological effects of clorazepate in man. Br J Clin Pharmacol 9:83–90, 1980

Lader M, Ron M, Petursson H: Computed axial brain tomography in long-term benzodiazepine users. Psychol Med 14:203–206, 1984

Ladewig D: Dependence liability of the benzodiazepines. Drug and Alcohol Abuse 13:139–149, 1984

Laegreid L, Olegard R, Wahlstrom J, et al: Abnormalities in children exposed to benzodiazepines in utero. Lancet 1:108–109, 1987

Landauer AA: Diazepam and traffic accidents. Br Med J 2:207, 1978

Landauer AA: Diazepam and driving ability. Med J Aust 1:624–626, 1981

Lasagna L: The Halcion story: trial by media. Lancet 1:815–816, 1980

Laughren TP, Battey YW, Greenblatt DJ: Chronic diazepam treatment in psychiatric outpatients. J Clin Psychiatry 43:461–462, 1982a

Laughren TP, Battey Y, Greenblatt DJ, et al: A controlled trial of diazepam withdrawal in chronically anxious outpatients. Acta Psychiatr Scand 65:171–179, 1982b

Laux G, Puryear DA: Benzodiazepines—misuse, abuse, and dependency. Am Fam Physician 30:139–147, 1984

Lawton MP, Cahn B: The effects of diazepam (Valium) and alcohol on psychomotor performance. J Nerv Ment Dis 136:550–554, 1963

Leifer ED, Goldman J, Finnegan LP: Prevalence and implications of multi-drug abuse in a population of methadone-maintained women. Natl Inst Drug Abuse Res Monogr Ser 43:323–328, 1983

Levy AB: Delirium and seizures due to abrupt alprazolam withdrawal: case report. J Clin Psychiatry 45:38–39, 1984

Liljequist R, Linnoila M, Mattila MJ: Effect of diazepam and chlorpromazine on memory functions in man. Eur J Clin Pharmacol 13:339–343, 1978

Liljequist R, Palva E, Linnoila M: Effects on learning and memory of 2-week treatments with chlordiazepoxide lactam, N-desmethyldiazepam, oxazepam, and methyloxazepam, alone or in combination with alcohol. International Pharmacopsychiatry 14:190–198, 1979

Lin SC, Morse RM, Finlayson RE, et al: Abuse of benzodiazepines (letter). JAMA 261:2956, 1989

Linnoila M, Hakkinen S: Effects of diazepam and codeine, alone and in combination with alcohol, on simulated driving. Clin Pharmacol Ther 15:368–373, 1974

Linnoila M, Mattila MJ: Drug interaction on driving skills as evaluated by laboratory tests and by a driving simulator. Pharmako-Psychiatrie Neuro-Psychopharmakologie 6:127–132, 1973

Linnoila M, Viukari M: Efficacy and side effects of nitrazepam and thioridazine as sleeping aids in psychogeriatric in-patients. Br J Psychiatry 128:566–569, 1976

Linnoila M, Saario I, Maki M: Effect of treatment with diazepam or lithium and alcohol on psychomotor skills related to driving.

Eur J Pharmacol 7:337–342, 1973

Linnoila M, Liljequist R, Olkoniemi J, et al: Effect of alcohol and benzodiazepines on performance as related to personality characteristics: personality characteristics among healthy "placebo reactors" and nonreactors. Pharmako-Psychiatrie Neuro-Psychopharmakologie 10:246–253, 1977

Linnoila M, Erwin CW, Brendle A, et al: Pharmacodynamics and pharmacokinetics of diazepam in an abuser. Acta Pharmacologica et Toxicologica 47:75–77, 1980a

Linnoila M, Viukari M, Lamminsivu U, et al: Efficacy and side effects of lorazepam, oxazepam, and temazepam as sleeping aids in psychogeriatric inpatients. International Pharmacopsychiatry 15:129–135, 1980b

Lipsitz LA: Falls and syncope, in Geriatric Medicine. Edited by Rowe JW, Besdine RW. Boston, Little, Brown, 1988, pp 208–218

Lister RG: Amnesic action of benzodiazepines in man. Neurosci Biobehav Rev 9:87–94, 1985

Lister RG, File SE: The nature of lorazepam-induced amnesia. Psychopharmacology 83:183–187, 1984

Long DH, Eltringham RJ: Lorazepam as night sedation and premedication: a comparison with dichloralphenazone and papaveretum. Anaesthesia 32:649–653, 1977

Lucki I, Rickels K: Differential effects of the anxiolytic drugs diazepam and buspirone on memory. Psychopharmacology 89:555, 1986

Lucki I, Rickels K, Geller AM: Chronic use of benzodiazepines and psychomotor and cognitive test performance. Psychopharmacology 89:S55, 1986

Lucki I, Rickels K, Giesecke MA, et al: Differential effects of the anxiolytic drugs, diazepam and buspirone on memory function. Br J Clin Pharmacol 23:207–211, 1987

Lukas SE, Griffiths RR: Precipitated withdrawal by a benzodiazepine receptor agonist (Ro 15-1788) after 7 days of diazepine. Science 217:1161–1163, 1982

Lyndon RW, Russell JD: Benzodiazepine use in a rural general practice population. Aust N Z J Psychiatry 22:293–298, 1988

Mac DS, Kumar R, Goodwin DW: Anterograde amnesia with oral lorazepam. J Clin Psychiatry 46:137–138, 1985

Macdonald JB: The role of drugs in falls in the elderly. Clin Geriatr Med 1:621–636, 1985

MacKinnon GL, Parker WA: Benzodiazepine withdrawal syndrome: a literature review and evaluation. Am J Drug Alcohol Abuse 9:19–33, 1982

Maletzky BM, Klotter J: Addiction to diazepam. Int J Addict 2:95–

115, 1976

Malpas A, Legg NJ, Scott DF: Effects of hypnotics on anxious patients. Br J Psychiatry 124:482–484, 1974

Marks J: The Benzodiazepines: Use, Overuse, Misuse, Abuse. St. Leonard's House, Lancaster, United Kingdom, MTP Press, 1978

Marks J: Diazepam: the question of long-term therapy and withdrawal reactions. Drug Therapy 11 (Suppl):5–30, 1981

Marks J: Round table discussion, in The Benzodiazepines: From Molecular to Clinical Practice. Edited by Costa E. New York, Raven Press, 1983, pp 390–395

Marks J: Chronic anxiolytic treatment: benefit and risk, in Chronic Treatments in Neuropsychiatry. Edited by Kemali D, Racagni G. New York, Raven Press, 1985, pp 173–183

Marks J: Techniques of benzodiazepine withdrawal in clinical practice: a consensus workshop report. Medical Toxicology 3:324–333, 1988

Mattila MJ: Interactions of benzodiazepines on psychomotor skills. Br J Clin Pharmacol 18S:21S–26S, 1984

Mazzi E: Possible neonatal diazepam withdrawal: a case report. Am J Obstet Gynecol 129:586–587, 1977

McClish A: Diazepam as an intravenous induction agent for general anaesthesia. Canadian Anaesthetists Society Journal 13:562–575, 1966

McLeod DR, Hoehn-Saric R, Labib A, et al: Six weeks of diazepam treatment in normal women: effects of psychomotor performance and psychophysiology. J Clin Psychopharmacol 8:83–99, 1988

McNair DM: Anti-anxiety drugs and human performance. Arch Gen Psychiatry 29:609–617, 1973

McNicholas LF, Martin WR, Cherian S: Physical dependence on diazepam and lorazepam in the dog. J Pharmacol Exp Ther 226:783–789, 1983

Mead MG, Castleden CM: Psychotropic drugs, 4: confusion and hypnotics in demented patients. Journal of the Royal College of General Practitioners 32:763–765, 1982

Mellinger GD, Balter MB: Prevalence and patterns of use of psychotherapeutic drugs: results from a 1979 national survey of American adults, in Epidemiological Impact of Psychotropic Drugs. Edited by Tognoni G, Bellantuono C, Lader M. New York, Elsevier-North Holland, 1981, pp 117–135

Mellinger GD, Balter MB: Psychotherapeutic drugs: a current assessment of prevalence and patterns of use, in Society and Medication: Conflicting Signals of Prescribers and Patients. Edited by Morgan JP, Kagan DV. Lexington, KY, DC Heath and Co, 1983, pp 137–144

Mellinger GD, Balter MB, Parry HJ, et al: An overview of psychotherapeutic drugs, in Drug Use: Epidemiological and Sociological Approaches. Edited by Josephson E, Carroll EE. Hemisphere Publishing Corp, 1974, pp 333–365

Mellinger GD, Balter MB, Uhlenhuth EH: Anti-anxiety agents: duration of use and characteristics of users in the USA. Curr Med Res Opin 8S:21–35, 1984a

Mellinger GD, Balter MB, Uhlenhuth EH: Prevalence and correlates of the long-term regular use of anxiolytics. JAMA 251:375–379, 1984b

Mellinger GD, Balter MB, Uhlenhuth EH: Insomnia and its treatment. Arch Gen Psychiatry 42:225–232, 1985

Mellor CS, Jain VK: Diazepam withdrawal syndrome: its prolonged and changing nature. Can Med Assoc J 127:1093–1096, 1982

Mendelson G: Withdrawal reactions after oxazepam. Lancet 2:565, 1978

Mendelson WB, Weingartner H, Greenblatt DJ, et al: A clinical study of flurazepam. Sleep 5:350–360, 1982

Miller F, Whitcup S: Benzodiazepine use in psychiatrically hospitalized elderly patients. J Clin Psychopharmacol 6:384–385, 1986

Miller JD, Cisin IH, Gardner KH, et al: National Survey on Drug Abuse: Main Findings 1982. DHHS Publication (ADM) 83-1263. Rockville, MD, US Public Health Service, 1983

Miller LG, Greenblatt DJ, Barnhill JG, et al: Benzodiazepines' receptor binding of triazolobenzodiazepines in vivo: increased receptor number with low-dose alprazolam. J Neurochem 49:1595–1601, 1987a

Miller LG, Greenblatt DJ, Paul SM, et al: Benzodiazepine receptor occupancy in vivo: correlation with brain concentrations and pharmacodynamic actions. J Pharmacol Exp Ther 240:516–522, 1987b

Miller LG, Greenblatt DJ, Barnhill JG, et al: Chronic benzodiazepine administration, I: tolerance is associated with benzodiazepine receptor downregulation and decreased gamma-aminobutyric acid receptor function. J Pharmacol Exp Ther 246:170–176, 1988

Minter R, Murray GB: Diazepam withdrawal: a current problem in recognition. J Fam Pract 7:1233–1235, 1978

Misra PC: Nitrazepam (Mogadon) dependence. Br J Psychiatry 126:81–82, 1975

Missen AW, Cleary WT, Eng L, et al: Diazepam, alcohol, and drivers. N Z Med J 87:275–277, 1978a

Missen AW, Cleary WT, Eng L, et al: Prescription drugs, alcohol, and road fatalities. N Z Med J 88:418–419, 1978b

Mitler MM, Carskadon MA, Phillips RL, et al: Hypnotic efficacy of teenagers: long-term sleep evaluation. Br J Clin Pharmacol 8:63–68, 1979

Morgan HG, Bouluois J, Burns-Cox C: Addiction to prednisone. Br Med J 2:93–94, 1973

Morgan K: Effect of low-dose nitrazepam on performance in the elderly. Lancet 1:516, 1982

Morgan K, Oswald I: Anxiety caused by a short-life hypnotic. Br Med J 284:942, 1982

Morgan LK: Diazepam and awareness. Med J Aust 2:617–618, 1969

Moskowitz H, Smiley A: Effects of chronically adminstered buspirone and diazepam on driving related skills performance. J Clin Psychiatry 43:45–55, 1982

Murphy SM, Owen RT, Tyrer PJ: Withdrawal symptoms after six weeks' treatment with diazepam. Lancet 2:1389, 1984

Nagy A: Long-term treatment with benzodiazepines: theoretical, ideological, and practical aspects. Acta Psychiatr Scand [Suppl] 76S:47–55, 1987

Nelson RC: Estimates of benzodiazepine use, doses, and duration of use; data on seizures and other reported withdrawal. Denominator of exposure—How many individuals are exposed to benzodiazepines (unpublished manuscript). Washington, DC, US Food and Drug Administration, 1987

Neuteboom W, Zweipfenning PGM: Driving and the combined use of drugs and alcohol in the Netherlands. Forensic Sci Int 25:93–104, 1984

Nicholson AN, Spencer MB: Psychological impairment and low-dose benzodiazepine treatment. Br Med J 285:99, 1982

Nikaido AM, Ellinwood EH, Heatherly D, et al: Differential CNS effects of diazepam in elderly adults. Pharmacol Biochem Behav 27:273–281, 1987

Nikaido AM, Ellinwood EH, Heatherly D, et al: Age-related increase in CNS sensitivity to benzodiazepine as assessed by task difficulty. Psychopharmacology (in press)

Nolan L, O'Malley K: Patients, prescribing, and benzodiazepines. Eur J Clin Pharmacol 35:225–229, 1988

Noyes R, Clancy J, Coryell WH, et al: A withdrawal syndrome after abrupt discontinuation of alprazolam. Am J Psychiatry 142:114–116, 1985

Noyes R, Perry PJ, Crowe RR, et al: Seizures following the withdrawal of alprazolam. J Nerv Ment Dis 174:50–52, 1986

Noyes R, DuPont RL, Pecknold JC, et al: Alprazolam in panic

disorder and agoraphobia: results from a multicenter trial, II: patient acceptance, side effects, and safety. Arch Gen Psychiatry 45:423–428, 1988a

Noyes R, Garvey MJ, Cook BL, et al: Benzodiazepine withdrawal: a review of the evidence. J Clin Psychiatry 49:382–389, 1988b

Oblowitz H, Robins AH: The effect of clobazam and lorazepam on the psychomotor performance of anxious patients. Br J Clin Pharmacol 16:95–99, 1983

O'Brien CP, Woody GE: Sedative-hypnotics and antianxiety agents, in Psychiatry Update: American Psychiatric Association Annual Review, Vol 5. Edited by Frances AJ, Hales RE. Washington, DC, American Psychiatric Press, 1986, pp 186–199

O'Hanlon JF, Haak TW, Blaauw GJ, et al: Diazepam impairs lateral position control in highway driving. Science 217:70–81, 1982

Olajide D, Lader M: Depression following withdrawal from long-term benzodiazepine use: a report of four cases. Psychol Med 14:937–940, 1984

Orzack MH, Cole JO, Dessain E, et al: A comparative study of the abuse liability of alprazolam, lorazepam, diazepam, methaqualone, and placebo, in Agenda and Abstracts for Panic Disorder Biological Research Workshop, Washington, DC, April 14–16, 1986

Oswald I: Withdrawal symptoms and rebound anxiety after six week course of diazepam (letter). Br Med J 290:1827, 1985

Owen RT, Tyrer P: Benzodiazepine dependence: a review of the evidence. Drugs 25:385–398, 1983

Pagano RR, Conner JT, Bellville JW, et al: Lorazepam, hyoscine, and atropine as iv surgical premedicants. Br J Anaesth 50:471–475, 1978

Palva ES, Linnoila M: Effect of active metabolites of chlordiazepoxide and diazepam, alone or in combination with alcohol, on psychomotor skills related to driving. Eur J Clin Pharmacol 13:345–350, 1978

Palva ES, Linnoila M, Saario I, et al: Acute and subacute effects of diazepam on psychomotor skills: interaction with alcohol. Acta Pharmacologica et Toxicologica 45:257–264, 1979

Pandit SK, Heisterkamp DV, Cohen PJ: Further studies of the anti-recall effect of lorazepam: a dose-time effect. Anesthesiology 45:495–500, 1976

Patterson J: Alprazolam dependency: use of clonazepam for withdrawal. South Med J 81:830–831, 836, 1988

Paul SM: Clinical implications of the GABA hypothesis, in Neuroscience Update. Kalamazoo, MI, Upjohn Company, 1987

Pearce C: The respiratory effects of diazepam supplementation of spinal anaesthesia in elderly males. Br J Anaesth 46:439–441, 1974

Pecknold JC, McClure DJ, Fleury D, et al: Benzodiazepine withdrawal effects. Prog Neuropsychopharmacol Biol Psychiatry 6:517–522, 1982

Pecknold JC, Swinson RP, Kuch K, et al: Alprazolam in panic disorder and agoraphobia: results from a multicenter trial, III: discontinuation effects. Arch Gen Psychiatry 45:429–436, 1988

Peel HW, Perrigo BJ, Mikhael NZ: Detection of drugs in saliva of impaired drivers. J Forensic Sci 29:185–189, 1984

Peet M, Moonie L: Abuse of benzodiazepines. Br Med J 1:714, 1977

Perera KMH, Powell T, Jenner FA: Computerized axial tomographic studies following long-term use of benzodiazepines. Psychol Med 17:775–777, 1987a

Perera KMH, Tulley M, Jenner FA: The use of benzodiazepines among drug addicts. Br J Addict 82:511–515, 1987b

Petersen RC: Influence of diazepam (Valium) on human learning and memory processes. Federation Proceedings 35:308, 1976

Petersen RC, Ghoneim MM: Diazepam and human memory: influence on acquisition, retrieval, and state-dependent learning. Prog Neuropsychopharmacol Biol Psychiatry 4:81–89, 1980

Petursson H, Lader MH: Withdrawal from long-term benzodiazepine treatment. Br Med J 235:643–645, 1981a

Petursson H, Lader MH: Withdrawal reaction from clobazam. Br Med J 282:1931–1932, 1981b

Petursson H, Lader MH: Psychological impairment and low-dose benzodiazepine treatment. Br Med J 285:815–816, 1982

Pevnick JS, Jansinski DR, Haertzen CA: Abrupt withdrawal from therapeutically administered diazepam: report of a case. Arch Gen Psychiatry 35:995–998, 1978

Pfefferbaum B, Butler P, Mullins D, et al: Two cases of benzodiazepine toxicity in children. J Clin Psychiatry 48:450–452, 1987

Photiades C, Lokantzis NA, Kaprinis G, et al: The effect of psychotropic drugs on learning ability. International Journal of Neurology 10:282–287, 1975

Pinsker H, Suljaga-Petchel K: Use of benzodiazepines in primary-care geriatric patients. J Am Geriatr Soc 32:595, 1984

Pishkin V, Fishkin SM, Shurley JT, et al: Cognitive and psychophysiologic response to doxepin and chlordiazepoxide. Compr Psychiatry 19:171–178, 1978

Pomara N, Stanley B, Block R, et al: Adverse effects of single therapeutic doses of diazepam on performance in normal geriatric subjects: relationship to plasma concentrations. Psychopharmacology 84:342–346, 1984

Pomara N, Stanley B, Block R, et al: Increased sensitivity of the elderly to the central depressant effects of diazepam. J Clin Psychiatry 46:185–187, 1985

Poser W, Poser S, Rosher D, et al: Do benzodiazepines cause cerebral atrophy? Lancet 1:715, 1983

Poswillo D: Intravenous amnesia for dental and oral surgery. N Z Dent J 63:265–270, 1967

Power KG, Jerrom DWA, Simpson RJ, et al: Controlled study of withdrawal symptoms and rebound anxiety after six week course of diazepam for generalized anxiety. Br Med J 290: 1246–1248, 1985

Preskorn SH, Denner LJ: Benzodiazepines and withdrawal psychosis. JAMA 237:36–38, 1977

Preston KL, Griffiths RR, Stitzer ML, et al: Diazepam and methadone interactions in methadone maintenance. Clin Pharmacol Ther 36:534–541, 1984

Public Citizen Health Research Group: Drug induced tranquility. Health Letter 3:6–8, 1987

Ramster D, Barber AJ, Deb A, et al: A policy on benzodiazepines (letter). Lancet 2:1406, 1987

Raskin M, Bradfor T: Methylphenidate (Ritalin) abuse and methadone maintenance. Diseases of the Nervous System 36:9–12, 1975

Ratna L: Addiction to temazepam. Br Med J 282:1837, 1981

Ray WA, Griffin MR, Schaffner W, et al: Psychotropic drug use and the risk of hip fracture. N Engl J Med 316:363–369, 1987

Redmond DE: Alprazolam: high-dose kinetics in primates, in Agenda and Abstracts for Panic Disorder Biological Research Workshop, Washington, DC, April 14–16, 1986

Reidenberg MM, Levy M, Warner H, et al: Relationship between diazepam dose, plasma level, age, and central nervous system depression. Clin Pharmacol Ther 23:371–374, 1978

Relkin R: Death following withdrawal of diazepam. NY State J Med 66:1770–1772, 1966

Rementeria JL, Bhatt K: Withdrawal symptoms in neonates from intrauterine exposure to diazepam. J Pediatr 90:123–126, 1977

Rickels K: Are benzodiazepines over-used and abused? Br J Clin Pharmacol 11:715–835, 1981

Rickels K: Benzodiazepines in the treatment of anxiety: North American experiences, in The Benzodiazepines: From Molecular Biology to Clinical Practice. Edited by Costa E. New York, Raven Press, 1983, pp 295–310

Rickels K: Clinical management of benzodiazepine dependence. Br Med J 291:1649, 1985

Rickels K: Determinants of chronic benzodiazepine use and dependence. Paper presented at the Annual Meeting of the American College of Neuropsychopharmacology, San Juan, Puerto Rico, December 1987

Rickels K, Schweizer E: Current pharmacotherapy of anxiety and panic, in Psychopharmacology: The Third Generation in Progress. Edited by Meltzer HY. New York, Raven Press, 1987, pp 1193–1203

Rickels K, Case WG, Diamond L: Relapse after short-term drug therapy in neurotic outpatients. International Pharmacopsychiatry 15:186–192, 1980

Rickels K, Case G, Downing RW, et al: Long-term diazepam therapy and clinical outcome. JAMA 250:767–771, 1983

Rickels K, Case WG, Winokur A, et al: Long-term benzodiazepine therapy: benefits and risks. Psychopharmacol Bull 20:608–615, 1984

Rickels K, Case WG, Downing RW, et al: Indications and contraindications for chronic anxiolytic treatment: is there tolerance to the anxiolytic effect? in Chronic Treatments in Neuropsychiatry. Edited by Kemali D, Racagni G. New York, Raven Press, 193–204, 1985

Rickels K, Case G, Downing RW, et al: One-year follow-up of anxious patients treated with diazepam. J Clin Psychopharmacol 6:32–36, 1986a

Rickels K, Case WG, Schwiezer E, et al: Low-dose dependence in chronic benzodiazepine users: a preliminary report of 119 patients. Psychopharmacol Bull 22:407–415, 1986b

Rickels K, Morris R, Mauriello R, et al: Brotizolam, a triazolothienodiazepine, in insomnia. Clin Pharmacol Ther 40:293–299, 1986c

Rickels K, Fox IL, Greenblatt DJ: Clorazepate and lorazepam: clinical improvement and rebound anxiety. Am J Psychiatry 145:312–317, 1988a

Rickels K, Schweizer E, Case WG, et al: Benzodiazepine dependence withdrawal severity and clinical outcome: effects of personality. Psychopharmacol Bull 24:415–420, 1988b

Rickels K, Schweizer E, Csanalosi I, et al: Long-term treatment of anxiety and risk of withdrawal: prospective comparison of clorazepate and buspirone. Arch Gen Psychiatry 45:444–450, 1988c

Ries RK, Roy-Byrne PP, Ward NG, et al: Carbamazepine treatment for benzodiazepine withdrawal. Am J Psychiatry 146:536–537, 1989

Rifkin A, Quitkin F, Klein DF: Withdrawal reaction to diazepam.

JAMA 236:2172–2173, 1976

Roache JD, Griffiths RR: Comparison of triazolam and pentobarbital: performance impairment, subjective effects, and abuse liability. J Pharmacol Exp Ther 234:120–133, 1985

Robinson GM, Sellers CM: Diazepam withdrawal seizures. Can Med Assoc J 126:944–945, 1982

Rodrigo EK, King MB, Williams P: Health of long-term benzodiazepine users. Br Med J 296:603–606, 1988

Roehrs T, Zorick FJ, Sicklesteel JM, et al: Effects of hypnotics on memory. J Clin Psychopharmacol 3:310–313, 1983

Roehrs T, Lamphere J, Paxton C, et al: Temazepam's efficacy in patients with sleep onset insomnia. Br J Clin Pharmacol 17:691–696, 1984a

Roehrs T, McLenaghan A, Koshorek G, et al: Amnesic effects of lormetazepam. Psychopharmacology 1S:165–172, 1984b

Romney DM, Angus WR: A brief review of the effects of diazepam on memory. Psychopharmacol Bull 20:313–316, 1984

Rosenberg HC, Chiu TH: Decreased ^{3}H-diazepam binding is a specific response to chronic benzodiazepine treatment. Life Sci 24:803–808, 1979

Rosenberg HC, Chiu TH: Tolerance during chronic benzodiazepine treatment associated with decreased receptor binding. Eur J Pharmacol 70:453–460, 1981

Rosenberg HC, Chiu TH: Nature of functional tolerance produced by chronic flurazepam treatment in the cat. Eur J Pharmacol 81:357–365, 1982

Rosenberg HC, Smith S, Chiu TH: Benzodiazepine-specific and nonspecific tolerance following chronic flurazepam treatment. Life Sci 32:279–285, 1983

Roth T, Hartse KM, Saab PG, et al: The effects of flurazepam, lorazepam, and triazolam on sleep and memory. Psychopharmacology 70:231–237, 1980

Roth T, Roehrs R, Wittig R, et al: Benzodiazepines and memory. Br J Clin Pharmacol 18S:45–49, 1984

Saario I: Effect of hypnotics or psychotropic drugs and alcohol on psychomotor skills. Psychiatr Fenn 8:131–144, 1977

Saario I, Linnoila M: Effect of subacute treatment with hypnotics, alone or in combination with alcohol, on psychomotor skills related to driving. Acta Pharmacologica et Toxicologica 38:382–392, 1976

Saario I, Linnoila M, Mittila MJ: Modification by diazepam or thioridazine of the psychomotor skills related to driving: a subacute trial in neurotic out-patients. Br J Clin Pharmacol 3:843–848, 1976

Salkind MR, Silverstone T: The clinical and psychometric evaluation of flurazepam. Br J Clin Pharmacol 2:223–226, 1975

Salkind MR, Hanks GW, Silverstone JT: Evaluation of the effects of clobazam, a 1,5 benzodiazepine, on mood and psychomotor performance in clinically anxious patients in general practice. Br J Clin Pharmacol 7S:113–118, 1979

Salzman C: Benzodiazepine habituation and withdrawal. Family Practice Recertification 6S:39–47, 1984

Salzman C: Benzodiazepines for the treatment of disorders other than anxiety and insomnia. Paper presented at the Annual Meeting of the Association for Advancement of Neuroscience, Rome, Italy, September 1988

Salzman C: Treatment with anti-anxiety agents, in Treatments of Psychiatric Disorders, Vol 3. Washington, DC, American Psychiatric Association, 1989, pp 2036–2051

Salzman C, Kochansky GE, Shader RI, et al: Chlordiazepoxide-induced hostility in a small group setting. Arch Gen Psychiatry 31:401–405, 1974

Salzman C, Kochansky GE, Shader RI, et al: Is oxazepam associated with hostility? Diseases of the Nervous System 36:30–32, 1975

Salzman C, Shader RI, Greenblatt DJ, et al: Long versus short half-life benzodiazepines in the elderly: kinetics and clinical effects of diazepam and oxazepam. Arch Gen Psychiatry 40: 293–297, 1983

Salzman C, Glassman R, Fisher J, et al: Improvement in memory after benzodiazepine discontinuance in elderly nursing home residents: a pilot study (unpublished manuscript), 1989

Scarone S, Strambi LF, Cazlo CL: Effects of two dosages of chlordesmethyldiazepam on mnestic-information processes in normal subjects. Clin Ther 4:184–191, 1981

Scharf MB, Khosla N, Lysaght R, et al: Anterograde amnesia with oral lorazepam. J Clin Psychiatry 44:362–364, 1983

Scharf MB, Khosla N, Brocker N, et al: Differential amnestic properties of short- and long-acting benzodiazepines. J Clin Psychiatry 45:51–53, 1984

Scharf MB, Saskin P, Fletcher K: Benzodiazepine-induced amnesia: clinical laboratory findings. J Clin Psychiatry (Monograph) 5:14–17, 1987

Schmauss C, Krieg JC: Enlargement of cerebrospinal fluid spaces in long-term benzodiazepine users. Psychol Med 17:869–873, 1987

Schmauss C, Apelt S, Emrich HM: The seeking and linking potentials of alprazolam. Am J Psychiatry 145:128, 1988

Schneider LS, Syapin PJ, Pawluczyk S: Seizures following triazolam withdrawal despite benzodiazepine treatment. J Clin Psychiatry 48:418–419, 1987

Schneider-Helment D: Why low-dose benzodiazepine dependent insomniacs can't escape their sleeping pills. Acta Psychiatr Scand 78:706–711, 1988

Schöpf J: Unusual withdrawal symptoms after long-term administration of benzodiazepines. Nervenarzt 52:288–292, 1981

Schöpf J: Withdrawal phenomena after long-term administration of benzodiazepines: a review of recent investigations. Pharmacopsychiatry 16:1–8, 1983

Schuckit MA, Morrissey ER: Drug abuse among alcoholic women. J Clin Psychiatry 136:607–611, 1979

Schweizer E, Rickels K: Failure of buspirone to manage benzodiazepine withdrawal. Am J Psychiatry 143:1590–1592, 1986

Schweizer E, Rickels K, Zavodnick S, et al: Clinical and medication status at one-year follow-up after maintenance treatment of panic disorder. Paper presented at the Annual Meeting of the Collegium Internationale Neuro-Psychopharmacologicum, Munich, 1988

Selig JW Jr: A possible oxazepam abstinence syndrome. JAMA 198: 951–952, 1966

Seppala T, Aranko K, Mattilla MJ, et al: Effects of alcohol on buspirone and lorazepam actions. Clin Pharmacol Ther 32: 201–207, 1982

Shader RI, Greenblatt DJ: Clinical implications of benzodiazepine pharmacokinetics. Am J Psychiatry 134:652–656, 1977

Shader RI, Greenblatt DJ: Triazolam and anterograde amnesia: all is not well in the Z-zone. J Clin Psychopharmacol 3:273, 1983

Shader RI, Dreyfuss D, Gerrein JR, et al: Sedative effects and impaired learning and recall following single oral doses of lorazepam. Clin Pharmacol Ther 39:526–529, 1986

Sheehan DV: One-year follow-up of patients with panic disorder and withdrawal from long-term antipanic medications, in Agenda and Abstracts for Panic Disorder Biological Research Workshop, Washington, DC, April 14–16, 1986

Sheehan D: Benzodiazepines in panic disorder and agoraphobia. J Affect Disord 13:169–181, 1987

Shur E, Petursson H, Checkley S, et al: Long-term benzodiazepine administration blunts growth hormone response to diazepam. Arch Gen Psychiatry 40:1105–1108, 1983

Skegg DCG, Richards SM, Doll R: Minor tranquillisers and road accidents. Br Med J 1:917–919, 1979

Smiley A, Moskowitz H: Effects of long-term administration of buspirone and diazepam on driver steering control. Am J Med

80(Suppl 3B):22–29, 1986

Smith BD, Nacev V: Drug usage as determined under conditions of anonymity and high questionnaire return rate. Int J Addict 13:725–736, 1978

Smith DE, Wesson DR: Benzodiazepine dependency syndromes, in The Benzodiazepines: Current Standards for Medical Practice. Edited by Smith DE, Wesson DR. Lancaster, United Kingdom, MTP Press, 1985, pp 235–248

Soni SD, Smith ED, Shah A: Hall of lorazepam withdrawal seizures: role of predisposition and multidrug therapies. Int Clin Psychopharmacol 1:165–169, 1986

Spinweber CL, Johnson LC: Effects of triazolam (0.5 mg) on sleep, performance, memory, and arousal threshold. Psychopharmacologia 76:5–12, 1982

Starmer GA, Bird KD: Investigating drug-ethanol interactions. Br J Clin Pharmacol 18S:27–35, 1984

Stewart RB, Salem RB, Springer PK: A case report of lorazepam withdrawal. Am J Psychiatry 137:1113–1114, 1980

Stitzer ML, Griffiths RR, McLellan AJ, et al: Diazepam use among methadone maintenance patients: pattern and dosages. Drug Alcohol Depend 8:189–199, 1981

Stovner J, Endresen R: Diazepam in intravenous anaesthesia. Lancet 2:1298, 1965

Subhan Z, Harrison C, Hindmarch I: Alprazolam and lorazepam single and multiple-dose effects on psychomotor skills and sleep. Eur J Clin Pharmacol 29:709–712, 1986

Tansella ZC, Tansella M, Lader M: A comparison of the clinical and psychological effects of diazepam and amylobarbitone in anxious patients. Br J Clin Pharmacol 7:605–611, 1979

Tedeschi G, Griffiths AN, Smith AT, et al: The effect of repeated doses of temazepam and nitrazepam on human psychomotor performance. Br J Clin Pharmacol 20:361–367, 1985

Terhune KW, Fell JC: The Role of Alcohol, Marijuana, and Other Drugs in the Accidents of Injured Drivers. National Highway Traffic Safety Administration Technical Report DOT HS-806 181. Washington, DC, US Department of Transportation, 1982

Tien AY, Gujavarty KS: Seizure following withdrawal from triazolam. Am J Psychiatry 142:1516–1517, 1985

Tinetti ME, Speechley M, Ginter SF: Risk factors for falls among elderly persons living in the community. N Engl J Med 319:1701–1707, 1988

Tyrer P: Benzodiazepine dependence and propranolol. Pharmaceutical Journal 225:158–160, 1980a

Tyrer P: Lorazepam withdrawal seizures. Lancet 1:151, 1980b

Tyrer P, Murphy S: The place of benzodiazepines in psychiatric practice. Br J Psychiatry 151:719–723, 1987

Tyrer P, Seivewright N: Identification and management of benzodiazepine dependence. Postgrad Med J 60S:41–46, 1984

Tyrer P, Rutherford D, Huggett T: Benzodiazepine withdrawal symptoms and propranolol. Lancet 1:520–522, 1981

Tyrer P, Owen R, Dowling S: Gradual withdrawal of diazepam after long-term therapy. Lancet 1:1402–1406, 1983

Uhde TW, Kellner CH: Cerebral ventricular size in panic disorder. J Affective Disord 12:175–178, 1987

Uhlenhuth EH, Balter MB, Mellinger GD, et al: Symptoms checklist syndromes in the general population. Arch Gen Psychiatry 40:1167–1173, 1983

Uhlenhuth EH, Balter MB, Mellinger GD, et al: Anxiety disorders: prevalence and treatment. Curr Med Res Opin 8S:37–46, 1984

Uhlenhuth EH, De Wit H, Balter MB: Risks and benefits of long-term benzodiazepine use. J Clin Psychopharmacol 8:161–167, 1988

Valentour JC, McGee BS, Edwards RP, et al: A survey of drug use among impaired drivers in Virginia. Med Leg Bull 29:1–7, 1980

Vine J, Watson TR: Incidence of drug and alcohol intake in road traffic accident victims. Med J Aust 1:612–615, 1983

Vital-Herne J, Brenner R, Lesser M: Another case of alprazolam withdrawal syndrome. Am J Psychiatry 142:1515, 1985

Voltato NA, Batcha KJ, Olson SC: Comment: alprazolam withdrawal (letter). Drug Intell Clin Pharm 21:754–755, 1987

Vyas I, Carney MWP: Diazepam withdrawal fits (letter). Br Med J 4:44, 1975

Weddington WW, Carney AC: Alprazolam abuse during methadone maintenance therapy (letter). JAMA 257:3363, 1987

Wetherell A: Individual and group effects of 10 mg diazepam on drivers' ability, confidence, and willingness to act in a gap-judging task. Psychopharmacology 63:259–267, 1979

Whitcup SM, Miller F: Unrecognized drug dependence in psychiatrically hospitalized elderly patients. J Am Geriatr Soc 35:297–301, 1987

White JM, Clardy DO, Graves MH, et al: Testing for sedative-hypnotic drugs in the impaired driver: a survey of 72,000 arrests. Clinical Toxicology 18:945–957, 1981

Wilbur R, Kulvik AV: Abstinency syndrome from therapeutic doses of oxazepam. Can J Psychiatry 28:298–301, 1983

Williams AF, Peat MA, Crouch DJ, et al: Drugs in fatally injured young male drivers. Public Health Rep 100:19–25, 1986

Willumeit HP, Ott H, Neubert W, et al: Alcohol interaction of lormetazepam, mepindolol sulphate, and diazepam, measured by performance on the driving simulator. Pharmacopsychiatria 17:36–43, 1984a

Willumeit HP, Ott H, Neubert W: Simulated car driving as a useful technique for the determination of residual effects and alcohol interaction after short- and long-acting benzodiazepines. Psychopharmacology 1S:182–192, 1984b

Wilson D: Experience with drugs and driving in Queensland, Australia. Med Sci Law 25:2–10, 1985

Winokur A, Rickels K, Greenblatt DJ, et al: Withdrawal reaction from long-term, low-dosage administration of diazepam. Arch Gen Psychiatry 37:101–105, 1980

Winstead DK, Anderson A, Eilers K, et al: Diazepam on demand: drug-seeking behavior in psychiatric inpatients. Arch Gen Psychiatry 30:349–351, 1974

Wiseman SM, Spencer-Peet J: Prescribing for alcoholics: a survey of drugs taken prior to admission to an alcoholism unit. Practitioner 229:88–89, 1985

Wittenborn JR: Effects of benzodiazepines on psychomotor performance. Br J Clin Pharmacol 7:615–765, 1979

Wittenborn JR: Behavioral toxicity of psychotropic drugs. J Nerv Ment Dis 168:171–176, 1980

Wolf B, Iguchi MY, Griffiths RR: Sedative/tranquilizer use and abuse: incidence, pattern and preference in alcoholics, in Problems of Drug Dependence. Edited by Harris LS. Washington, DC, U.S. Department of Health and Human Services, 1989

Woodhouse EJ: The prevalence of drugs in fatally injured drivers: alcohol, drugs, and traffic safety, in Proceedings of the Sixth International Conference on Alcohol, Drugs, and Traffic Safety, Toronto, September 1974. Edited by Israelstam S, Lambert S. Toronto, Addiction Research Foundation of Ontario, 1975, pp 147–158

Woods JH: Benzodiazepine dependence studies in animals: an overview. Drug Development Research 1S:77–81, 1982

Woods JH, Katz JL, Winger G: Abuse liability of benzodiazepines. Pharmacol Rev 39:251–419, 1987

Woods JH, Katz JL, Winger G: Use and abuse of benzodiazepines. JAMA 260:3476–3480, 1988

Woody GE, Mintz J, O'Hare K, et al: Diazepam use by patients in a methadone program: how serious a problem? Journal of Psychedelic Drugs 7:373–379, 1975a

Woody GE, O'Brien CP, Greenstein R: Misuse and abuse of diazepam: an increasingly common medical problem. Int J Addict

10:843–848, 1975b

Zipursky RB, Baker RW, Zimmer B: Alprazolam withdrawal delirium unresponsive to diazepam: case report. J Clin Psychiatry 46: 344–345, 1985

Additional Readings

The following sources were used as background for the Task Force Report, but were not directly cited.

Bartholomew AA, Reynolds WS: Four cases of progressive drug abuse. Med J Aust 54:653–657, 1967

Baskin SI, Esdale A: Is chlordiazepoxide the rational choice among benzodiazepines? Pharmacotherapy 2:110–119, 1982

Beaudry P, Chouinard G, Annable L: Clonazepam in the treatment of patients with recurrent panic attacks. J Clin Psychiatry 47:83–85, 1986

Bitnum S: Possible effect of chlordiazepoxide on the fetus (letter). Can Med Assoc J 100:351, 1969

Blackwell B: Benzodiazepines: drug abuse and data abuse. Psychiatric Opinion 16:10–37, 1979

Bliding A: Effects of different rates of absorption of two benzodiazepines on subjective and objective parameters: significance of clinical use and risk of abuse. Eur J Clin Pharmacol 7:201–211, 1974

Bond AJ, Lader M: After-effects of sleeping drugs, in Psychopharmacology of Sleep. Edited by Wheatley D. New York, Raven, 1981, pp 177–197

Bowes HA: The role of diazepam (Valium) in emotional illness. Psychosomatics 6:36–40, 1965

Braestrup C, Neilsen M, Squires RF: No changes in rat benzodiazepine receptors after withdrawal from continuous treatment with lorazepam and diazepam. Life Sci 135–143, 1979

Browne TR: Benzodiazepines in human seizure disorders, in Pharmacology of Benzodiazepines. Edited by Usdin E, Skolnick P, Tallman J, et al. London, Macmillan, 1983, pp 329–337

Burke GW, Anderson CWG: Response to Librium in individuals with a propensity for addiction: a pilot study. Journal of the Louisiana State Medical Society 114:58–60, 1962

Buschke H: Selective reminding for analysis of memory and learning. Journal of Verbal Learning and Verbal Behavior 12:543–550, 1973

Busto U, Kaplan HL, Sellers EM: Benzodiazepine-associated emergencies in Toronto. Am J Psychiatry 137:224–227, 1980

Cannizzaro G, Nigito S, Provenzano PM, et al: Modification of depressant and disinhibitory action of flurazepam during short-term treatment in the rat. Psychopharmacologia 26:173–184, 1972

Catalan J, Gath D, Bond A, et al: The effects of non-prescribing of anxiolytics in general practice, II: factors associated with outcome. Br J Psychiatry 144:603–610, 1984

Catalan J, Gath D, Edmonds G, et al: The effects of non-prescribing of anxiolytics in general practice, I: controlled evaluation of psychiatric and social outcome. Br J Psychiatry 144:593–602, 1984

Chan AWK: Effects of combined alcohol and benzodiazepine: a review. Drug Alcohol Depend 13:315–341, 1984

Chiu TH: Reduced diazepam binding following chronic benzodiazepine treatment. Life Sci 21:1153–1157, 1978

Chiu TH, Rosenberg HC: GABA receptor-mediated modulation of ^{3}H-diazepam binding in rat cortex. Eur J Pharmacol 56:337, 1979

Ciraulo D, Olsen D: Pharmacokinetic response and tolerance studies of alprazolam in patients with panic disorder, in Agenda and Abstracts for Panic Disorder Biological Research Workshop, Washington, DC, April 14–16, 1986

Clift AD: Factors leading to dependence on hypnotic drugs. Br Med J 3:614–617, 1972

Clift AD: A general practice study of dependence on some non-barbiturate hypnotic drugs, in Sleep Disturbance and Hypnotic Drug Dependence. Edited by Clift AD. Amsterdam, Excerpta Medica, 1975, pp 97–105

Clift AD: Prediction of the dependence-prone patient—a general practice investigation: personality or drug effect, in Sleep Disturbance and Hypnotic Drug Dependence. Edited by Clift AD. Amsterdam, Excerpta Medica, 1975, pp 107–153

Clinthorne JK, Cisin IH, Balter MB, et al: Changes in popular attitudes and beliefs about tranquilizers. Arch Gen Psychiatry 43:527–532, 1986

Cohen LS, Rosenbaum JF: Clonazepam: New uses and potential problems. J Clin Psychiatry 48S:50–55, 1987

Cole JO: Medication and seclusion and restraint. McLean Hospital Journal 10:37–53, 1985

Cole JO, Haskell DS, Orzack MH: Problems with the benzodiazepines: an assessment of the available evidence. McLean Hosp J 6:46–74, 1981

Committee on the Review of Medicines: Systematic review of the benzodiazepines. Br Med J 280:910–912, 1980

Conell LJ, Berlin RM: Withdrawal after substitution of a short-acting for a long-acting benzodiazepine. JAMA 250:2838–2840, 1983

Cook L, Sepinwall J: Behavioral analysis of the effects and mechanisms of action of benzodiazepines, in Mechanisms of Action of the Benzodiazepines. Edited by Costa E, Greengard P. New York, Raven Press, 1975

Cooper SA, Anthony JE, Mopsik E, et al: A technique for investigating the intensity and duration of human psychomotor impairment after intravenous diazepam. Oral Surg Oral Med Oral Pathol 45:493–502, 1978

Csernansky JG, Hollister L: Withdrawal reaction following therapeutic doses of benzodiazepines. Hospital Formulary 18:900–902, 1983

Daly RJ, Kane FJ: Two severe reactions to benzodiazepine compounds. Am J Psychiatry 122:577–578, 1965

Danger ahead! Valium. Vogue, February 1975, pp 152–153

Dawson GW, Jue SG, Brogden RN: Alprazolam—a review of its pharmacodynamic properties and efficacy in the treatment of anxiety and depression. Drugs 27:132–147, 1984

DeAngelis L, File SE: Acute and chronic effects of three benzodiazepines in the social interaction anxiety test in mice. Psychopharmacology 64:127, 1979

De Buck R: Clinical experience with lorazepam in the treatment of neurotic patients. Curr Med Res Opin 1:291–295, 1973

Dehlin O, Bjornson G: Triazolam as a hypnotic for geriatric patients. Acta Psychiatr Scand 67:290–296, 1983

De Wit H, Johanson CE, Uhlenhuth EH, et al: The effects of two nonpharmacological variables on drug preference in humans, in Problems of Drug Dependence, 1982. Edited by Harris LS. NIDA Research Monograph 43. Washington, DC, US Department of Health and Human Services, 1983, pp 251–257

Dilsaver SC, Greden JF: Antidepressant withdrawal-induced activation (hypomania and mania): mechanism and theoretical signficance. Brain Research Reviews 7:29–48, 1984

diStefano P, Case KR, Colello GD, et al: Increased specific binding of ^{3}H-diazepam in rat brain following chronic diazepam administration. Cell Biol Int Rep 3:163–167, 1979

Divoll M, Greenblatt DJ, Hermann R, et al: Absolute bioavailability of oral and intramuscular diazepam: effects of age and sex. Anesth Analg 62:1–8, 1983

Drury VWM: Benzodiazepines: a challenge to rational researching. J R Coll Gen Pract 35:86–88, 1985

Dundee JW, Haslett WHK, Keilty SR, et al: Studies of drugs given before anaesthesia, XX: diazepam-containing mixtures. Br J Anaesth 42:143–150, 1970

Dunlop DM, Henderson TL, Inch RS: A survey of 17,301 prescriptions on form EC 10. Br Med J 1:292–295, 1952

Dunnell K, Cartwright A: Medicine Takers, Prescribers, and Hoarders. London, Routledge and Kegan Paul, 1972

Eakins WA, Faloon D: The profile of the suspect drunk-in-charge driver in the Belfast area. Ulster Med J 46:32–37, 1977

Edwards DS, Hahn CP, Fleishman EA: Evaluation of laboratory methods for the study of driver behavior: the relation between simulator and street performance, in AIR Report R69 7. Washington, DC, American Institutes for Research, 1969

Elie R, Lamontagne Y: Alprazolam and diazepam in the treatment of generalized anxiety. J Clin Psychopharmacol 4:125–129, 1984

Emmett-Oglesby MW, Spencer DG, Elmesallamy F, et al: The pentylenetetrazole model of anxiety detects withdrawal from diazepam in rats. Life Sci 33:161–168, 1983

Epstein FB: Fatal benzodiazepine toxicity? (letter). Am J Emerg Med 5:472, 1987

Essig CF: Addiction to nonbarbiturate sedative and tranquilizing drugs. Clin Pharmacol Ther 5:334–343, 1964

Essig CF: Newer sedative drugs that can cause states of intoxication and dependence of barbiturate type. JAMA 196:714–717, 1966

Ewing JA, Bakewell WE: Diagnosis and management of depressive drug dependence. Am J Psychiatry 123:909–917, 1967

Fawcett JA, Kravits HM: Alprazolam: pharmacokinetics, clinical efficacy, and mechanisms of action. Pharmacotherapy 2:243–254, 1982

Ferrara SD, Castagna F, Tedeschi L: Alcohol, drugs, and road accidents in Northeast Italy: preliminary report, in Alcohol, Drugs, and Traffic Safety. Proceedings of the Eighth International Conference on Alcohol, Drugs, and Traffic Safety, June 1980. Edited by Goldberg L. Stockholm, Sweden, Almqvish Wicksell, 1980, pp 315–327

Finkle BS, McCloskey KL, Goodman LS: Diazepam and drug associated deaths: a survey in the United States and Canada. JAMA 242:429–434, 1979

Food and Drug Administration Center for Drug and Biologics: Adverse behavioral reactions attributed to triazolam. Washington, DC, Department of Health and Human Services, 1987

Fox R: Abuse of benzodiazepines. Lancet 2:681–682, 1978

Fyer AJ: Alprazolam withdrawal in patients with panic, in Agenda and Abstracts for Panic Disorder Biological Research Workshop, Washington, DC, April 14–16, 1986

Garattini S, Mussini E, Randall LO (eds): The Benzodiazepines. New York, Raven Press, 1973

Garbus SB, Weber MA, Priest RT, et al: The abrupt discontinuation of antihypertensive treatment. J Clin Pharmacol 19:476–486, 1979

Gelbke HB, Schlicht HJ, Schmidt G: Haufigkeit positiver diazepam, befunde in blutproben alkoholisierter verkehrsteilnehmer. Z Rechtsmed 80:319–328, 1978

Gershon S, Eison AS: Anxiolytic profiles. J Clin Psychiatry 44:45–56, 1983

Ghadirian AM, Gauthier S, Wong T: Convulsions in patients abruptly withdrawn from clonazepam while receiving neuroleptic medication (letter). Am J Psychiatry 144:686, 1987

Ghoneim MM, Korttilia K, Chiang CK, et al: Diazepam effects and kinetics in Caucasians and Orientals. Clin Pharmacol Ther 29:749–756, 1981

Glatt MM: The abuse of barbiturates in the United Kingdom. Bull Narc 14:19–38, 1962

Glatt MM: Benzodiazepines (letter). Br Med J 2:444, 1967

Glatt MM: Benzodiazepine abuse in alcoholics. Lancet 2:1205, 1971

Glauzer FL, Smith R: Physiologic and biochemical abnormalities in self-induced drug overdosage. Arch Intern Med 135:1468–1473, 1975

Goldberg ME, Manian AA, Efron DH: A comparative study of certain pharmacologic responses following acute and chronic administrations of chlordiazepoxide. Life Sci 6:481–491, 1967

Gonzalez JP, McCulloch AJ, Nichols PJ, et al: Subacute benzodiazepine treatment: observations on behavioral tolerance and withdrawal. Alcohol Alcohol 19:325–332, 1984

Gray JA, Holt L, McNaughton N: Clinical implications of the experimental pharmacology of the benzodiazepines, in The Benzodiazepines: From Molecular Biology to Clinical Practice. Edited by Costa E. New York, Raven Press, 1983, pp 147–172

Greenblatt DJ, Shader RI: Pharmacokinetic aspects of anxiolytic drug therapy. Can J Neurol Sci 7:269–270, 1980

Greenblatt DJ, Shader RI, Koch-Weser J: Psychotropic drug use in the Boston area. Arch Gen Psychiatry 32:518–521, 1975

Greenblatt DJ, Woo E, Allen MD, et al: Rapid recovery from massive diazepam overdose. JAMA 240:1872–1874, 1978

Greenblatt DJ, Laughren TP, Thomas P, et al: Plasma diazepam and desmethyldiazepam concentrations during long-term diaze-pam therapy. Br J Clin Pharmacol 11:35–40, 1981

Greenblatt DJ, Divoll M, Abernethy DR, et al: Clinical pharmacokinetics of the newer benzodiazepines. Clin Pharmacokinet 8:233–252, 1983

Greenblatt DJ, Divoll M, Abernethy DR, et al: Reduced clearance of triazolam in old age: relation to antipyrine oxidizing capacity. Br J Clin Pharmacol 15:303–309, 1983

Greenblatt DJ, Shader RI, Divoll M, et al: Adverse reactions to triazolam, flurazepam, and placebo in controlled clinical trials. J Clin Psychiatry 45:192–195, 1984

Greist JH, Jefferson JW, Marks IM: Anxiety and Its Treatment. Washington, DC, American Psychiatric Press, 1986

Guile LA: Rapid habituation to chlordiazepoxide ("Librium"). Med J Aust 50:56–57, 1963

Haefely W: Benzodiazepine receptors: summary and commentary, in Pharmacology of Benzodiazepines. Edited by Usdin E, Skolnick P, Tallman JF, et al. London, Macmillan, 1983, pp 175–184

Hallstrom C, Lader M: Benzodiazepine withdrawal phenomena. International Pharmacopsychiatry 16:235–244, 1981

Hallstrom C, Lader M: The incidence of benzodiazepine dependence in long-term users. Journal of Psychiatric Treatment and Evaluation 4:293–296, 1982

Hartelius H, Larsson AK, Lepp M, et al: A controlled long-term study of flunitrazepam, nitrazepam, and placebo, with special regard to withdrawal effects. Acta Psychiatr Scand 58:1–15, 1978

Hartse KM, Roth T, Piccione PM, et al: Rebound insomnia (letter). Science 208:423–424, 1980

Hasday JD, Karch FE: Benzodiazepine prescribing in a family medicine center. JAMA 246:1321–1325, 1981

Hawthorne JW, Zabora JR, Dlugoff BC: Out-patient detoxification of patients addicted to sedative-hypnotics and anxiolytics. Drug Alcohol Depend 9:143–151, 1982

Hayashki T, Higashki T, Kadota K: Three cases of chronic chlordiazepoxide intoxication and their withdrawal symptoms. J Clin Psychiatry 16:77–83, 1974

Hearings Before the Subcommittee on Health and Scientific Research of the Senate Committee on Human Resources: The Use and Abuse of Valium, Librium, and Other Benzodiazepine Tranquilizers. 97th Congress, 1st Session, 1979

Heel R, Brogden RN, Speight TM, et al: Temazepam. Drugs 21:321–340, 1981

Helman CG: "Tonic," "fuel," and "food": social and symbolic aspects of the long-term use of psychotropic drugs. Soc Sci Med 15B:521–533, 1981

Herrygers EJ: Drug abuse and overdosage information. NDA, July 10, 1987

Hillestad L, Hansen T, Melsom H: Diazepam metabolism in normal man, II: serum concentration and clinical effect after oral administration and cumulation. Clin Pharmacol Ther 16:485–489, 1974

Hollister LE: Benzodiazepines 1980: a look at the issues. Psychosomatics 21S:4–8, 1980

Hollister LE: Benzodiazepine dependence said to be relatively rare. Clinical Psychiatry News 9:24, 1981

Hollister LE: Dependence on benzodiazepines, in Benzodiazepines: A Review of Research Results, 1980. Edited by Saraza SI, Ludford JP. Natl Inst Drug Abuse Res Monogr Ser 33:70–83, 1981

Hollister LE: Management of the anxious patient prone to drug abuse. J Clin Psychiatry 42:35–39, 1981

Hollister LE: Drug tolerance, dependence, and abuse. Current Concepts, October 1985

Hollister LE, Glazener FS: Withdrawal reactions for meprobamate alone and combined with promazine: a controlled study. Psychopharmacologia 1:336–341, 1960

Hollister LE, Bennett JL, Kimbell I Jr, et al: Diazepam in newly admitted schizophrenics. Diseases of the Nervous System 24:746–750, 1963

Hoogland DR, Misya TS, Bousquet WF: Metabolism and tolerance studies with chlordiazepoxide 2-14C in the rat. Toxicol Appl Pharmacol 9:116–123, 1960

Hrbek J, Komenda S, Birkas O, et al: On the acute effect of some drugs on the higher nervous activity in man, part IX: amitriptyline (50 mg), nortriptyline (50 mg), diazepam (10 mg). Acta Univ Palacki Olomuc Fac Med 47:655–667, 1967

Hrbek J, Komenda S, Macakova J, et al: On the acute effect of some drugs on the higher nervous activity in man, part XIII: diazepam (10 mg), alimemazine (25 mg), meprobamate (1,000 mg). Acta Univ Palacki Olomuc Fac Med 49:307–323, 1968

Hrbek J, Komenda S, Macakova J, et al: The acute effect of diazepine derivatives on the higher nervous activity in man. Aggressologie 19:189–191, 1978

Jacoby RJ, Levy R, Dawson JM: Computerized tomography in the elderly, I: the normal population. Br J Psychiatry 136:249–255, 1980

Jauhar P: Non-opiate abuse amongst opiate addicts, in The Misuse of Psychotropic Drugs. Edited by Murray R, Ghodse H, Harris C, et al. London, Gaskell Publishers, 1981 pp 71–73

Jencks SF: Recognition of mental distress and diagnosis of mental disorder in primary care. JAMA 253:1903–1907, 1985

Johanson CE, Kilgore K, Uhlenhuth EH: Assessment of dependence potential of drugs in humans using multiple indices. Psychopharmacology 81:144–149, 1983

Johnson LC, Spinweber CL: Benzodiazepine activity: the sleep electroencephalogram and daytime performance. Clin Neuropharmacol 8S:101S–111S, 1985

Johnson LC, Spinweber CL, Seidel WF, et al: Sleep spindle and delta changes during chronic use of a short-acting and a long-acting benzodiazepine hypnotic. Electroencephalogr Clin Neurophysiol 55:662–667, 1983

Johnson LC, Mitler MM, Dement WC: Comparative hypnotic effects of flurazepam, triazolam, and placebo: another look. J Clin Psychopharmacol 5:180–181, 1985

Jones DM, Lewis MJ, Spriggs TLB: The effects of low doses of diazepam on human performance in group administered tasks. Br J Clin Pharmacol 6:333–337, 1978

Kalant H, LeBlanc AE, Gibbons RJ: Tolerance to, and dependence on, some non-opiate psychotropic drugs. Pharmacol Rev 23: 135–191, 1971

Kales A: Drug dependency: investigations of stimulants and depressants. Ann Intern Med 70:591–614, 1969

Kales A, Preston TA, Tan TL, et al: Hypnotics and altered sleep dream patterns. Arch Gen Psychiatry 23:211–218, 1970

Kales A, Bixler EO, Soldatos CR, et al: Quazepam and temazepam: effects of short- and intermediate-term use and withdrawal. Clin Pharmacol Ther 39:345–352, 1986

Kales A, Soldatos CR, Bixler EO, et al: Diazepam: effects on sleep and withdrawal phenomena. J Clin Psychopharmacol 8:340–346, 1988

Kanto J, Iisalo E, Lehtinen V, et al: The concentrations of diazepam and its metabolites in the plasma after an acute and chronic administration. Psychopharmacologia 36:123–131, 1974

Kellet JM: The benzodiazepine bonanza (letter). Lancet 2:9–64, 1974

Kemper N, Posser W, Posser S: Benzodiazepine dependence: addiction potiential of the benzodiazepines is greater than previously assumed. Dtsch Med Wochenschr 105:1707–1712, 1980

Kendall MJ: Hazards of abrupt withdrawal of drugs. Prescribers Journal 18:25–34, 1978

Kielholz P, Goldberg L, Obersteg JM, et al: Strassenverkehr, tranquilizer, und alkohol. Dtsche Med Wochenschr 92:1525–1531, 1967

Killian GA, Holzman PS, Davis JM, et al: Effects of psychotropic medication on selected cognitive and perceptual measures. J Abnorm Psychol 93:58–70, 1984

Koenig W, Ruther E, Filipiak B: Psychotropic drug utilization patterns in a metropolitan population. Eur J Clin Pharmacol 32:43–51, 1987

Koeppen D: Review of clinical studies on clobazam: proceedings of a symposium on clobazam. Br J Clin Pharmacol 7:139S–150S, 1979

Koeppen D: Memory and benzodiazepines: animal and human studies with 1,4-benzodiazepines and clobazam (1,5-benzodiazepine). Drug Development Research 4:555–566, 1984

Kohn R, White KL: Health Care: An International Study. Report of the World Health Organization/International Collaborative Study of Medical Care Utilization. Oxford, Oxford University Press, 1976

Korttila K, Linnoila M: Recovery and skills related to driving after intravenous sedation: dose-response relationship with diazepam. Br J Anaesth 47:457–463, 1975

Kryspin-Exner K: Missbrauch von benzodiazepinderivaten be: alkhoholkranken. Br J Addict 61:283–292, 1966

Lader M: Benzodiazepines—the opium of the masses? Neuroscience 3:159–165, 1978

Lader M: Psychological effects of buspirone. J Clin Psychiatry 43:62–67, 1982

Lader M, Higgitt A: Management of withdrawal from benzodiazepines. International Drug Therapy Newsletter 21:21–23, 1986

Lader M, Olajide D: A comparison of buspirone and placebo in relieving benzodiazepine withdrawal symptoms. J Clin Psychopharmacol 7:11–15, 1987

Lader M, Petursson H: Benzodiazepine derivatives—side effects and dangers. Biol Psychiatry 16:1195–1201, 1981

Lamb RJ, Griffiths RR: Physical dependence on benzodiazepines: spontaneous and precipitated withdrawal syndromes in the baboon (abstract). Federation Proceedings 44:1636, 1985

Lapierre YD: Benzodiazepines withdrawal. Can J Psychiatry 26:93–95, 1981

Lapierre YD: Are all benzodiazepines clinically equivalent? Prog Neuropsychopharmacol Biol Psychiatry 7:641–646, 1983

Lapierre YD, Tremblay A, Gagnon A, et al: A therapeutic and discontinuation study of clobazam and diazepam in anxiety neurosis. J Clin Psychiatry 43:372–374, 1982

Larson E, Kukull WA, Buchner D, et al: Adverse drug reactions associated with global cognitive impairment in elderly persons. Ann Intern Med 107:169–173, 1987

Leppik IE, Derivan AT, Homan RW, et al: Double-blind study of lorazepam and diazepam in status epilepticus. JAMA 249: 1452–1454, 1983

Leysen JE, Gompel PV, Gommeren W: Down regulation of serotonin-S2 receptor sites in rat brain by chronic treatment with the serotonin-S2 antagonists: ritanserin and setoperone. Psychopharmacology 88:434–444, 1986

Liljequist R, Mattila MJ: Acute effects of temazepam and nitrazepam on psychomotor skills and memory. Acta Pharmacologica et Toxicologica 44:364–369, 1979

Lingjaerde O: Effects of the benzodiazepine derivative estozolam in patients with auditory hallucinations. Acta Psychiatr Scand 65:339–354, 1982

Linnoila M, Saario I, Olkoniemi J, et al: Effect of two weeks' treatment with chlordiazepoxide or flupenthixole, alone or in combination with alcohol on psychomotor skills related to driving. Arzneimittelforschung 25:1088–1092, 1975

Linnoila M, Erwin CW, Brendle A, et al: Psychomotor effects of diazepam in anxious patients and healthy volunteers. J Clin Psychopharmacol 3:88–96, 1983

Lippmann SB: Trazodone cardiac effects. International Drug Therapy Newsletter 20:29–32, 1985

Lister RG, File SE: Performance impairment and increased anxiety resulting from the combination of alcohol and lorazepam. J Clin Psychopharmacol 3:66–71, 1983

Litovitz T: Fatal benzodiazepine toxicity? the author replies (letter). Am J Emerg Med 5:472–473, 1987

Loke WH, Hinrichs JV, Ghoneim MM: Caffeine and diazepam: separate and combined effects on mood, memory, and psychomotor peformance. Psychopharmacology 87:344–350, 1985

Lucki I, Rickels K, Geller AM: Psychomotor performance following the long-term use of benzodiazepines. Psychopharmacol Bull 21:93–96, 1985

Lupolover R, Dazzi H, Ward J: Rebound phenomena: results of a 10 years' (1970–1980) literature review. International Pharmacopsychiatry 17:194–237, 1982

Manheimer DI, Mellinger GD, Balter MB: Psychotherapeutic drugs: use among adults in California. California Medicine 109:445–451, 1968

Manheimer DI, Davidson ST, Balter MB, et al: Popular attitudes and beliefs about tranquilizers. Am J Psychiatry 130:1246–1253, 1973

Marangos PJ, Crawley JN: Chronic benzodiazepine treatment increases [^{3}H]muscimol binding in mouse brain. Neuropharmacology 21:81–84, 1982

Margules DL, Stein L: Increase of "antianxiety" activity and tolerance of behavioral depression during chronic administration of oxazepam. Psychopharmacology 13:74–80, 1968

Marks J: The benzodiazepines—for good or evil. Neuropsychobiology 10:115–126, 1983

Mattila M, Aranko K, Seppala T: Acute effects of buspirone and alcohol and psychomotor skills. J Clin Psychiatry 43:56–60, 1982

Mattila M, Seppala T, Mattila MJ: Combined effects of buspirone and diazepam on objective and subjective tests of performance in healthy volunteers. Clin Pharmacol Ther 40:620–626, 1986

Mellinger GD, Balter MB, Uhlenhuth EH: A cross-national comparison of anti-anxiety/sedative drug use. Curr Med Res Opin 8S:5–19, 1984

Merz WA, Ballmer U: Symptoms of benzodiazepine withdrawal in untreated anxiety (abstract no. 131.2), in Abstract from the Fourth World Congress of Biological Psychiatry, Philadelphia, September 1985

Miller F, Nulsen J: Single case study. Diazepam (Valium) detoxification. J Nerv Ment Dis 167:637–638, 1979

Mitcheson M, Davidson J, Hawks D, et al: Sedative abuse by heroin addicts. Lancet 1:606–607, 1970

Mohler H, Sieghart W, Polc P, et al: Differential interaction of agonists and antagonists with benzodiazepine receptors, in Pharmacology of Benzodiazepines. Edited by Usdin E, Skolnick P, Tallman JF, et al. London, Macmillan, 1982, pp 63–70

Moire SJ, Sellers EM: Use of drugs with dependence liability. Can Med Assoc J 121:717–723, 1979

Mordell JS: The Prescription of the Pharmaceutical Survey. Washington, DC, American Council on Education, 1949

Muller C: The overmedicated society: forces in the marketplace for medical care. Science 176:488–492, 1972

Müller-Oerlinghausen B: Prescription and misuse of benzodiazepines in the Federal Republic of Germany. Pharmacopsychiatry 19:8–13, 1986

Murray J: Long-term psychotropic drug taking and the process of withdrawal. Psychol Med 11:853–858, 1981

Murray J, Dunn G, Williams P, et al: Factors affecting the consumption of psychotropic drugs. Psychol Med 11:551–560, 1981

Murray J, Williams P, Clare A: Health and social characteristics of long-term psychotropic drug takers. Soc Sci Med 16:1595–1598, 1982

Nathan RG, Robinson D, Cherek DR, et al: Alternative treatments for withdrawing the long-term benzodiazepine user: a pilot study. Int J Addict 21:195–211, 1986

Nicholson AN: Hypnotics: rebound insomnia and residual sequelae. Br J Clin Pharmacol 9:223–225, 1980

Nicholson AN: The use of short- and long-acting hypnotics in clinical medicine. Br J Clin Pharmacol 11:61S–69S, 1981

Nicholson AN, Stone BM, Spencer MB: Anxiety caused by a short-life hypnotic (letter). Br Med J 284:1785, 1982

Norman TR, Burrows GD: Plasma levels of benzodiazepine antianxiety drugs and clinical response, in Handbook of Studies on Anxiety. Edited by Burrows GD, Davies B (eds). Amsterdam, Elsevier, 1980

Northern Regional Health Authority: Benzodiazepine dependence and withdrawal. Newcastle upon Tyne, United Kingdom, Northern Regional Health Authority, April 1983 (Drugs Newsletter Supplement)

Ochs HR, Miller LG, Greenblatt DJ, et al: Actual versus reported benzodiazepine usage by medical outpatients. Eur J Clin Pharmacol 32:383–388, 1987

O'Hanlon JF: Driving performance under the influence of drugs: rationale for, and application of, a new test. Br J Clin Pharmacol 18:121S–129S, 1984

Oswald I: Dependence upon hypnotic and sedative drugs, in Contemporary Psychiatry. Edited by Silverman T, Barraclough B. Ashford, Great Britain, Headly, 1976, pp 272–277

Oswald I, Priest RG: Five weeks to escape the sleeping-pill habit. Br Med J 2:1093–1095, 1965

Pakes EE, Brodgen RN, Heel RC, et al: Triazolam. Drugs 22:81–110, 1981

Palmer GC: Use, overuse, misuse and abuse of benzodiazepines. Ala J Med Sci 15:383–392, 1978

Parish PA: The prescribing of psychotropic drugs in general practice. J R Coll Gen Pract 21:1S–77S, 1971

Parry HJ, Balter MB, Mellinger GD, et al: National patterns of psychotherapeutic drug use. Arch Gen Psychiatry 28:769–783, 1973

Paul SM, Skolnick P: Comparative neuropharmacology of antianxiety drugs. Pharmacol Biochem Behav 17:37–41, 1982

Pecknold JC, Swinson RP: Prospective alprazolam/placebo discontinuation—Canadian study, in Agenda and Abstracts for Panic

Disorder Biological Research Workshop. Washington, DC, April 14–16, 1986

Pegram V, Hude P, Linton P: Chronic use of triazolam: the effect of the sleep patterns of insomniacs. J Int Med Res 8:224–231, 1980

Perera KMH, Jenner FA: Some characteristics distinguishing high- and low-dose users of benzodiazepines. Br J Addict 82:1329–1334, 1987

Perry PJ, Stambaugh RL, Tsuang MT, et al: Sedative-hypnotic tolerance testing and withdrawal comparing diazepam to barbiturates. J Clin Psychopharmacol 1:289–296, 1981

Petursson H, Lader M: Benzodiazepine dependence. Br J Addict 76:133–145, 1981

Petursson H, Lader M: Benzodiazepine withdrawal syndrome, in New Psychiatric Syndromes: DSM-III and Beyond. Edited by Akhtar S. New York, Jason Aronson, 1983, pp 177–190

Petursson H, Lader M: Benzodiazepine tolerance and withdrawal syndrome, in Advances in Human Psychopharmacology. Edited by Burrows GD, Werry JS. Greenwich, CT, JAI Press, 1984, pp 89–119

Petursson H, Lader M: Dependence on tranquilizers. New York, Oxford University Press, 1984

Petursson H, Shur E, Checkley S, et al: A neuroendocrine approach to benzodiazepine tolerance and dependence. Br J Clin Pharmacol 11:526–528, 1981

Petursson H, Bhattacharya SK, Glover V, et al: Urinary monoamine oxidase inhibitor and benzodiazepine withdrawal. Br J Psychiatry 140:7–10, 1982

Petursson H, Gudjonsson GH, Lader MH: Psychometric performance during withdrawal from long-term benzodiazepine treatment. Psychopharmacology 81:345–349, 1983

Pitts WM, Fann WE, Sajadi C, et al: Alprazolam in older depressed inpatients. J Clin Psychiatry 44:213–215, 1983

Quitkin FM, Rifkin A, Kaplan J, et al: Phobic anxiety syndrome complicated by drug dependence and addiction. Arch Gen Psychiatry 27:159–162, 1972

Raferty EB: Cardiovascular drug withdrawal syndromes: a potential problem with calcium antagonists? Drugs 28:371–374, 1984

Randall LO, Heise GA, Schallek W, et al: Pharmacological and clinical studies on Valium, a new psychotherapeutic agent of the benzodiazepine class. Current Therapeutic Research 3: 405–425, 1961

Rangno RE, Langlois S: Comparison of withdrawal phenomena

after propranolol, metoprolol and pindolol. Br J Clin Pharmacol 13S:345–351, 1982

Redmond DE: New directions in panic disorder treatment discontinuation, in Agenda and Abstracts for Panic Disorder Biological Research Workshop. Washington, DC, April 14–16, 1986

Rickels K: Benzodiazepines: use and misuse, in Anxiety: New Research and Changing Concepts. Edited by Klein DF, Rabkin J. New York, Raven Press, 1981, pp 1–26

Rickels K: Alprazolam in the management of anxiety, in Drug Treatment of Neurotic Disorders—Focus on Alprazolam. Edited by Lader MH, Davies HC. Edinburgh, Churchill Livingstone, 1985, pp 84–93

Rickels K, Gingrich RL, Morris RJ, et al: Triazolam in insomniac family practice patients. Clin Pharmacol Ther 18:315–324, 1975

Rickels K, Csanalosi I, Greisman P, et al: A controlled clinical trial of alprazolam for the treatment of anxiety. Am J Psychiatry 140:82–85, 1983

Rickels K, Csanalosi I, Chung H, et al: Buspirone, clorazepate, and withdrawal, in Program and Abstracts of the 138th Annual Meeting of the American Psychiatric Association, Dallas, Texas, May 1985, pp 18–24

Robinson GM, Sellers EM, Janecek E: Barbiturate and hypnosedative withdrawal by a multiple oral phenobarbital loading technique. Clin Pharmacol Ther 30:71–76, 1981

Ryan GP, Boisse NR: Benzodiazepine tolerance, physical dependence and withdrawal: electrophysiological study of spinal reflex functions. J Pharmacol Exp Ther 231:464–471, 1984

Sabey BE: A review of drinking and drug taking in road accidents in Great Britain, in TRRL Supplementary Report 441. Crawthorne, England, Department of the Environment, Department of Transport, 1978, pp 1–9

Samson Y, Bernuau J: Cerebral uptake of benzodiazepine measured by positron emission tomography in hepatic encephalopathy. N Engl J Med 414, 1987

Sandler R: Benzodiazepines for anxiety (letter). Lancet 2:1273, 1987

Scharf MB, Hirschowitz J, Woods M, et al: Lack of amnestic effects of clorazepate on geriatric recall. J Clin Psychiatry 46:518–520, 1985

Schutz E: Toxicology of clobazam. Br J Clin Pharmacol 7S:33–35, 1979

Schweizer E, Rickels K, Zavodnick S, et al: Clinical and medication status at one year follow-up after maintenance treatment of panicdisorder. Paper presented at CINP Congress, Munich, Germany, August 1988

Schweizer E, Case WG, Rickels K: Benzodiazepine dependence and withdrawal in elderly patients. Am J Psychiatry 146:529–531, 1989

Shader RI, Greenblatt DJ, Salzman C, et al: Benzodiazepines: safety and toxicity. Diseases of the Nervous System 36:23–26, 1975

Skegg DC, Doll R, Perry J: Use of medicine in general practice. Br Med J 1:1561–1563, 1977

Slater J: Suspected dependence on chlordiazepoxide hydrochloride (Librium) (letter). Can Med Assoc J 95:416, 1966

Smith AJ: Self-poisoning with drugs: a worsening situation. Br Med J 4:157–159, 1972

Smith DE, Wesson DR: Benzodiazepine dependency syndromes. J Psychoactive Drugs 15:85–95, 1983

Snaith RP: Benzodiazepines on trial (letter). Br Med J 288:1379, 1984

Squires RF, Benson DI, Braestrup C, et al: Some properties of brain specific benzodiazepine receptors: new evidence for multiple receptors. Pharmacol Biochem Behav 10:825–830, 1979

Steentoft A, Worm K, Christensen H: The frequency in the Danish population of benzodiazepines in blood samples received for blood ethanol determination for the period June 1978 to June 1979. J Forensic Sci Soc 25:435–443, 1985

Stitzer ML, Bigelow GE, Liebson IA, et al: Contingent reinforcement for benzodiazepine-free urines: evaluation of a drug abuse treatment intervention. J Appl Behav Anal 15:493–503, 1982

Suzdak PD, Glowa JR, Crawley JN, et al: A selective imidazobenzo-diazepine antagonist of ethanol in the rat. Science 234:1247, 1986

Syvalahti EKG, Kanto JH: Serum growth hormone, serum immuno-reactive insulin and blood glucose response to oral and intra-venous diazepam. Int J Clin Pharm 12:74–82, 1975

Tessler R, Stokes R, Pietras M: Consumer response to Valium. Drug Therapy 8:178–183, 1978

Thiebot MH, Soubrie P: Behavior pharmacology of the benzo-diazepines, in The Benzodiazepines. Edited by Costa E. New York, Raven Press, 1983, pp 67–92

Thompson T, Unna KR (eds): Predicting Dependence Liability of Stimulant and Depressant Drugs. Baltimore, University Park Press, 1977

Trickett S: Withdrawal from benzodiazepines. J R Coll Gen Pract 33:608, 1983

Tyrer P: The benzodiazepine bonanza. Lancet 2:709–710, 1974

Tyrer P: Dependence on benzodiazepines. Br J Psychiatry 137:576–577, 1980

Tyrer P: Benzodiazepines on trial. Br Med J 288:1101–1102, 1984

Vellucci SV, File SE: Chlordiazepoxide loses its anxiolytic action with long-term treatment. Psychopharmacology 62:61–65, 1979

Viscott DS: Chlordiazepoxide and hallucinations. Arch Gen Psychiatry 19:370–376, 1968

Waldron I: Increased prescribing of Valium, Librium, and other drugs: an example of the influence of economic and social factors on the practice of medicine. Int J Health Serv 7:37–62, 1977

Weissman MM: Withdrawal after depression, in Agenda and Abstracts for Panic Disorder Biological Research Workshop, Washington, DC, April 14–16, 1986

Weppner GJ: The effect of benzodiazepine withdrawal on the dexamethasone suppression test. Acta Psychiatr Scand 77:232–234, 1988

White JM, Graves MH: The detection of sedative/hypnotic drugs in the impaired driver. J Chromatogr Sci 12:219–224, 1974

Williams P, Murray J, Clare A: A longitudinal study of psychotropic drug prescription. Psychol Med 12:201–206, 1982

Winter RM: In-utero exposure to benzodiazepine. Lancet 1:627, 1987

Wolf B, Ruether E: Drug abuse and dependence in psychiatric inpatients. Pharmacopsychiatria 18:37–39, 1985

World Health Organization, Expert Committee on Drug Dependence: Twentieth Report. WHO Tech Rep Ser, No. 551, 1974

World Health Organization Review Group: Use and abuse of benzodiazepines. Bull WHO 61:551–562, 1983

Yanagita T, Takahashi S: Dependence liability of several sedative-hypnotic agents evaluated in monkeys. J Pharmacol Exp Ther 185:307–316, 1973

Zingales IA: Diazepam metabolism during chronic medication: unbound fraction in plasma, erythrocytes and urine. J Chromatogr 75:55–78, 1973

Zisook S, De Vaul RA: Adverse behavioral effects of benzodiazepines. J Fam Pract 5:963–966, 1977

Index